Jim Gano

I'm

Not

Done

Yet ...

I'm

Not

Done

Yet ...

One Man's Journey from Cancer Survivor to *Thriver*

Jim Gano

2 3 4 5 6 7 8 9
First Printing

ISBN 978-0-9670591-3-6 (Paperback)
ISBN 978-0-9670591-5-0 (Hardback)
ISBN 978-0-9670591-4-3 (Ebook – Kindle)
ISBN 978-0-9670591-6-7 (downloadable audio file)

Library of Congress Number: 2024920274

Cover design by: Russ Zaborowski

Printed and published in the U.S.A. by

Phoenix Rising Publishing
A Division of GEI
15 Main Street – Suite 4
Flemington, NJ 08822

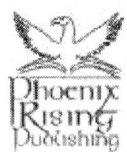

I'm Not Done Yet

Other books by Jim Gano (published as James Gano)

<u>Fiction</u>

The Student
The Player

Coming Soon
<u>Business</u>

The Action Plan

Dedication

This book is dedicated to my wife Carol. You will never know how much your love and guidance has meant to me both during my cancer journey, and our journey through life. I am hopeful we will have many more sunsets together.

I would be remiss if I didn't also dedicate this book to the wonderful doctors, nurses and staffs at Morristown Memorial Medical Center, in Morristown, New Jersey and at the John Theurer Cancer Center at Hackensack University Medical Center in Hackensack, New Jersey. I put my faith and life in your hands, and you gave both back to me. I will be forever grateful to everyone at these two institutions.

I also dedicate this to my kids and their wife and fiancée. Thanks for keeping it real, and not letting me get down during this process.

And to my friend and coach throughout this process, Suzanne Politi-Goldberg for taking my initial call and coaching me through this journey. You helped me in more ways than you will ever know and for that I love you, and I thank you.

Finally, to my three grandchildren, Brayden, Savannah and Peyton. You may never know what an important role you played in my recovery. Everything I went through and endured I did so I could watch you grow up. You bring Pop Pop joy every day with our video calls and occasional visits. As you'll hear in this story I am looking forward to Brayden's wedding.

Jim Gano

*"Life should not be a journey to the grave with the
intention of arriving safely in a pretty and well-
preserved body, but rather to skid in broadside in a
cloud of smoke, thoroughly used up, totally worn
out, and loudly proclaiming,
'Wow! What a ride!'"*

- Hunter S. Thompson

Introduction

This book is being written at the suggestion of several friends and even doctors who told me my story is unique and that I have a unique style of telling my story. One that hopefully you will find uplifting, motivational and inspirational. There will be times while reading this book when I might make you mad or sad, and that is not my intent. There will be times when you read this and you'll think, this guy is nuts, and you might be right.

This book is written with short chapters to introduce a subject, explain my approach to it, get you thinking about it, and then move on to the next. This is not, by any stretch of the imagination an all-encompassing how-to book on how to beat cancer, although I hope you or your loved one do just that. This is just one man's story, my story, of how I did, for now.

What do you mean for now? Well, my type of cancer I am told will recur at some point. At the time of this writing, I am in remission for two plus years and I can honestly say I am living my best life. I appreciate everything so much more than I ever took time to before. I don't take family members, especially my wife for granted. I appreciate everything and everyone so much more. I am more patient with people. A friend of mine once said "your being diagnosed with cancer is a gift, don't ever lose that." I'll explain what she meant in an upcoming chapter. But as you'll see, she makes perfect sense.

The front cover design has some special meaning to me. I own a classic car similar to the one pictured on the cover and I love taking it out for rides on the weekends and to the occasional car show. I pictured a man standing next to his car staring at a beautiful sunset. I did this because I have always loved that time of day and watching a beautiful sunset, in the mountains or at a beach. It is my way of putting the day to rest. I hope to see many more sunsets during my lifetime.

This book is written not only for the cancer patient, but also for their caregiver(s), their families and friends. Anyone who has ever dealt with someone who had cancer can benefit from reading this book. I sincerely hope it helps you as you navigate your way along the roads of your cancer journey. It is not an easy trip, and at times you may even feel lost along the way. Have faith, you can and will get through it, all of you, together. Most importantly be there for each other, help each other, encourage each other, listen to each other, love each other and most importantly share with each other what you are feeling.

The title of this book has special meaning to me, "I'm Not Done Yet." When I received my diagnosis, it suddenly put into perspective all that I had already done in my life, and more importantly, all I felt I had yet to do. I wasn't going to let something like cancer stop me from accomplishing all I wanted to do, neither should you. I call my dealing with cancer a "journey," not a fight. I truly had no idea where I was going on this journey, but I was willing to find out. In a sense, I did have to fight, and so will you, to find that inner resolve that will enable you to endure the medications, the pain, the needle sticks, the IV's, the ports, the chemo, the radiation, the surgeries (if applicable), the endless appointments, the insurance battles, etc. You will fight every day, but it is all part of the journey.

Make remission or cure your end point, your goal, your final destination, and work with your doctors, nurses, your family and friends, and others to get to that goal.

I wish you all the very best on your journey and pray for a successful outcome for anyone reading this.

Because like me, I hope ... you're not done yet.

My Story

This is my story. Many people who have known me for a long time, or just met me through my cancer journey encouraged me to write this book. Some said I was motivational, others said I was inspirational, one gentleman recently told me my story gave him hope as he is about half way through his own cancer journey. Still others told me that my story might help people as they embarked on their own journey with cancer. I don't know if any of that is true, but as someone who has written two books already, I figured I would give it a shot, my normal genre of writing is fiction. This story is not fiction. It is my story, and it is my truth.

I don't refer to my cancer as a battle or a fight, as some people do, but rather as a journey.

From my initial diagnosis, to chemo treatments, to a Stem cell transplant (SCT), to finally reaching remission and dealing with various hospitals, doctors and nurses, labs, etc., each event, appointment and interaction with everyone along the way was another step on my journey. A journey I continue every day since. You see once you have cancer and go through all that, it never really leaves you, but more on that in a later chapter.

It has taken me two years to finally put pen to paper, or in my case fingers to keyboard to write this. As I began several times, I asked myself who am I writing this for? Very few people except those closest to me would necessarily care to hear my story, but there might be others. Those looking for a light at the end of the tunnel or who need a little inspiration along the way from someone who "beat" cancer. So, I chose to write this book for them. I wrote it for the newly diagnosed individual. I wrote it for their loved ones who in many cases will become their caregivers, taking them to appointments, holding their hands and in general being there for them. I wrote it for those currently in treatment to encourage them to continue on in their fight. And selfishly, I wrote it for me. I did this to remind myself of all that I went through, regardless of how tough it was, so if I ever complain in the future all I'll have to do is look at this book and the rest will seem small.

Well, there is no better place to begin than the beginning so let's go there.

Back in early 2020 I had to go to my general practitioner for bloodwork for a routine physical. When I got the results, I noticed that a few of the markers were in the high range. I asked her about it and she asked me to come back to the office the following week for another blood test, this result was also abnormally high. We did this for two more weeks before she finally called me and said, *"I think you have a condition called Hemochromatosis and would like you to see a specialist at Morristown (NJ) Medical Center."*

The specialist she referred me to was a Hematology Oncologist. He reviewed the bloodwork and agreed with her assessment. Hemochromatosis is a condition in which your body stores too much iron in the blood. The treatment for this was that every two weeks I would have to go to the hospital and they would draw a pint of blood out of me. This procedure is similar to when you donate blood. Then we would watch the blood test results to see if there was any improvement and if the abnormally high numbers would come back down to the normal range.

After about four times of going to the hospital the doctor said I could stop and we would monitor my bloodwork every three months. I have always been a curious fellow so I re-reviewed the original blood tests. Then I consulted "Dr. Google" and would type in "What does a high result on ALT in bloodwork mean?" To which the Google machine would list 10–15 options. I did this for all of the abnormal blood markers, highs and lows, and a common denominator kept appearing, a cancer called Multiple Myeloma.

I mentioned this to my wife one night over dinner and she responded "how can you even say something like that? That is cancer." To be honest, she didn't actually respond, she yelled at me. To understand my wife, you have to know that she has spent her entire career in cancer research and worked on teams that brought three very successful chemotherapy drugs to market for her company. Out of college she completed a Medical Technologist program in addition to being a Phlebotomist. She knew how to interpret blood results. Still, she was not pleased that I had suggested the possibility I might have cancer.

A word of caution here regarding "Dr. Google." Be careful what you read and how you interpret it. It can be very scary, and you will think you are dying of everything when you simply have the common cold. An upcoming chapter is titled "trust, but verify," and that is some great advice when researching symptoms on the internet. The problem with the internet is that it is filled with false information, or outdated information, and as a result you could send your mind spinning into areas you don't want to go.

Everything was rolling along as we entered 2021 and I finally scheduled a surgery for July that I had been putting off for too long to have my right knee replaced. Keep in mind this was in the middle of the COVID-19 era. For one month before the surgery, I went to physical therapy three times a week to strengthen my leg so that when I came home from the surgery, I would be one step (pun intended) ahead in my recovery.

About four days before the surgery something gave way in my back. It felt like the worst muscle pull or spasm you could ever imagine. As I got out of bed one day I couldn't straighten up. I asked my wife to get me a cane behind a chair in our room that she had used when she had knee surgery a couple years prior and I pushed myself up with it.

I have a saying I use with my kids that goes *"power through it"* whenever anything gets tough. So that is what I did, I powered through the next few days at work and at home until it was surgery day. I had convinced myself it was just a strained muscle from the physical therapy I was doing. Finally, I had the surgery and the next day a nurse and physical therapist showed up at my house to begin my physical rehabilitation. Still, my back hurt like hell. Again, I blamed it on the initial physical therapy and a possible strained muscle.

After two weeks of in-home physical therapy, the knee was feeling better, the back was feeling worse. So, I did what any dummy would do and made an appointment with a chiropractor. For five weeks, three days a week he stimulated my back, tried to crack my back and neck with no relief then finally said he didn't think he could help me.

To explain how bad this had become, I could not lift the water pitcher from my refrigerator to the island counter three feet away. I had no strength.

Next! Next for me was going back to the physical therapist in their office. This was done mostly for my knee, but he was also concerned about my back and started giving me exercises for that, but nothing worked. A few weeks later he finally referred me to a pain management specialist at a local hospital.

Why are hospitals so big? Every department seemed to be at the opposite end of the hospital or parking lot and walking for me was becoming harder and harder with each passing day.

Finally, the pain management specialist ordered an X-Ray (of course 5 floors down and on the opposite side of the hospital). I rode in a wheelchair (thank God) and they took the X-Rays. I was wheeled back to his office and I could tell instantly by the look on his face and the tone of his voice this was no muscle pull. He said, "you have two compression fractures in your spine at T11 & T12." Basically, I had a broken back! I asked how this could happen and he laid out three scenarios 1). I weighed 600 pounds and my spine could not carry the weight. That was not the case. 2). I was 85 years old and Osteoporotic. I was only 60 at the time, so that was not the case either. Or 3). I had Multiple Myeloma a rare blood/bone cancer that was basically destroying my bones from the inside out. Now where did I hear that before? Oh yeah, that's what I thought I had a year earlier.

He arranged to have me fitted for a special back brace and referred me back to my general physician for follow-up. I joked with people that the brace was being used to put Humpty Dumpty back together again. The truth was I couldn't do anything without it. I could finally walk, and I could lift items up to ten pounds and I could sit a little while longer. Still the pain was unbearable. He mentioned a surgical procedure called a Kyphoplasty that could fix me if I was a suitable candidate.

When I went back to my family practice physician, she again ordered blood tests, but wasn't quite ready to confirm the pain management specialist's diagnosis. We did additional blood tests for three weeks when she finally called my wife and I at 7:30PM one night and said those words we all dread hearing, "*You have cancer. Specifically, you have Multiple Myeloma.*"

I should have been a doctor. I already have the horrible handwriting, but I made that diagnosis a year earlier. But, the thing with MM (that is how Multiple Myeloma patients refer to the disease) is that it can be "smoldering," or dormant for years and then one day it decides to awaken and unleash holy hell on your body.

I give my family physician all the credit in the world for basically saving my life. She never gave up and was always searching for definitive answers and a diagnosis she was confident in. Although inconvenient, she kept asking me to come to her office for more bloodwork. Those extra tests, and her tenacity are probably the reason I am alive today. If you don't have a doctor like her, find one. At the very least insist that your doctor exhaust all measures when searching for a diagnosis.

My doctor then referred me to see a doctor that specialized in blood disorders, a Hematology/Oncology doctor at Morristown Memorial Hospital, the same one I had met with during my Hemochromatosis diagnosis.

We met with him and based on the blood tests, a bone marrow biopsy, and a PET Scan he confirmed the diagnosis. This was on December 21, 2021.

It's funny how certain dates stick with you, this one will stick with me forever for two reasons. The first, is that is the date of my diagnosis, and the second is that was the date on the calendar on the wall of the Chipmunks Christmas album cover from the 1960's (I loved that album as a kid). Go ahead Google it, I'll wait.

And so began my cancer journey.

I have something to tell you ...

Let's go back for a minute. It was late 2021 and I was scheduled for a bone marrow biopsy (not fun) three days before Thanksgiving. Here, they say they numb you (and I'm sure they do) and jab a needle into your spine to remove spinal fluid and remove pieces of bone to be looked at under a microscope. It hurt, no two ways around it. And it also felt like the doctor was sucking my bone marrow out with a vacuum cleaner. I've now had two of these procedures and comparatively the first one was easy. The next one, not so much.

Just so you know as you read this, I have a friend who also has Multiple Myeloma and on occasion he asks me for advice and what to expect. As he puts it, "Give me the good, the bad and the ugly." That is what I am doing in this book for anyone who reads it. You may not like what you read, but if I said it doesn't hurt and you had this procedure and it did, you wouldn't like me very much. I also feel it is important for your caregiver and those around you to know what you are feeling throughout the process.

I enjoyed Thanksgiving with the family trying to think of football, family and anything but cancer. Not the easiest thing to do. On December first I followed up with the doctor and he said that the bone marrow biopsy confirmed the diagnosis of Multiple Myeloma and that there was about sixty percent involvement in my body. A PET scan was scheduled for December 20th to determine where the cancer was and if it had spread.

Three weeks. I now had to endure three weeks of not knowing how bad this was. Just go to work, come home, have dinner, watch TV. You know as if this all-consuming news wasn't real. The clock kept ticking and I was growing impatient to get this stuff (cancer) out of me. Finally, the 20th arrived and I lay on the table as best I could with two broken vertebrae in my back as this machine travelled up and down my body taking 3-D pictures of my insides.

Finally, I was done. Now I would just await the results which fortunately, I only had to wait one day for. The next day my wife and I met with the doctor and his nurse practitioner to review the films and plot the next steps.

That was when we finally received a confirmed and undeniable diagnosis of Multiple Myeloma. Fortunately, the cancer had not spread to any vital organs. It was nicely contained in my blood and bones. I guess they are vital too, but at least I would only be fighting one cancer and not two or three. I will say this, the PET scan is the coolest imaging I have ever seen of the human body. It was a 3-D image of my insides. The doctor could take the mouse and rotate the image front, back and sideways. I could see pins in my feet from a prior surgery, the knee replacement hardware, and a spinal cord stimulator that had been implanted years earlier. What I couldn't see was cancer in any vital organs or tumors on any bones and I was very relieved by that.

As for me, the doctor never said, "you have cancer." Instead, he said, "based on the bloodwork, bone marrow biopsy and PET scan that reveals you have sixty percent involvement in your bones, I am inclined to diagnose you with Multiple Myeloma."

What wonderful news to receive four days before Christmas. *Fa la la la la . . .*

When you receive this news, it is as if time somehow stops. For me there was no noise in the room. The doctor was talking, my wife was asking questions, I asked a few questions myself, but my mind which I thought had been prepared for this news suddenly stopped functioning, or so it seemed. I couldn't hear. My brain was doing its best to process this "official" diagnosis, but couldn't. I might have even shaken my head to clear the cobwebs as if I had just been punched in the nose and rejoined the conversation.

If you could have seen a tally counter connected to my brain you would have seen the numbers climb rapidly representing all the questions which were now occupying my brain. What surprised me was where were all these questions during the last three weeks? Was I that good at ignoring the possibility that I had cancer, or just in denial? At this point I didn't know and didn't care, I had to pay attention to the rest of this conversation.

I knew something was wrong all along, and I had been mentally preparing myself for what might come next, a cancer diagnosis. Still, having it confirmed in such a matter-of-fact manner caught me a little off-guard. If you ever start being tested for cancer my advice would be to begin to mentally prepare yourself for what is to come. Someone once told me "Expect the best, prepare for the worst." Good advice as it pertains to cancer.

After informing me of the diagnosis, he asked if I needed a minute to process this information and I said, "no." He asked "what do you mean, no?" I replied, "I have cancer. I get that, now I need to know what the next steps are." He looked at me and my wife and said, "Well, I will review your case and set you up with a chemotherapy regimen that will lead you up to a Stem cell transplant which I will refer you to another doctor who heads up the transplant team at Hackensack University Medical Center."

He mentioned a few chemotherapy drugs, cocktails or combinations if you will, that he could try based on all of my test results.

I said, "Okay when do we start?" He was taken aback by this and said, "We should be able to start by late January or early February." He wanted to review all of my results to see which 'chemo combo' he thought would achieve the best results. I said, "Do you have anything next week?" He replied, "That is Christmas week." I said, "I know, but I have cancer now, so I don't want to wait until February to get started, let's start now." I was seriously ready to begin right then.

I always close my business (Crown Trophy of Flemington, NJ) during the Christmas week, so I really didn't have anything else to do. I might be the only cancer patient who was actually happy to begin treatment, because to me it was a beginning to hopefully an end. An end to the pain, an end to the cancer, and a return to some sort of normalcy in our lives.

The doctor had obviously not encountered a patient like me before. There were no tears, no disbelief, no "why me?" just a "let's get this process started" attitude. He answered all of our remaining questions and said his Nurse Practitioner would call me later that day with the first available date. To which I told him the sooner the better. Later that afternoon she called, and I was scheduled to begin my chemotherapy regimen with my first appointment the following week on December 30th.

I was given steroids in the week leading up to the first infusion and on December 30th I arrived to begin a treatment regimen of Revlimid, Velcade, and Dexamethasone. This is probably one of the last times I will mention what drugs I was given because everyone's cancer and treatment regimen is different and their reaction to the drugs can be different too. Keep in mind this was all happening during the COVID-19 pandemic. My wife was allowed to be with me for that first visit, but after that I had to fly solo. So, while the poisons made their way out of the IV bags and into my arm I read books, listened to music and watched all the activity happening around me.

When I could, I would try to crack a few jokes with the nurses and technicians who were all super serious around the patients. I'm not sure if they appreciated my attempts at humor, but if it made them laugh, it put me at ease. We left that first treatment and I went home naively waiting for what I was sure was coming, the nausea and vomiting that you often hear about, but it never came. I was scheduled for sixteen chemo sessions but only needed twelve to move onto the next phase in my treatment, the Stem cell transplant. In fact, during my twelve chemo rounds I rarely got sick and only missed a day and a half of work. The nausea was ever present, but the anti-nausea meds they gave me helped me to mostly keep that under control.

As we drove home, in silence from receiving the diagnosis, I started to think about who I had to tell and how I had to tell them. Everybody knew I had been hurting with my back, but nobody knew why. I felt this might be an easy way to let them know that the compression fractures were caused by a cancer of the blood and bone.

This would not be easy, for me to say, or for them to hear. I decided not to tell anyone before Christmas, but after, or after dinner that night we would tell them. I really didn't want to ruin anyone's holiday with my diagnosis. I remember making a cryptic post on Facebook, intended for an audience of one and I hoped she got it.

The one person I hoped would see my message was a friend named Suzanne who had previously been a manager of mine at a company I worked for some twenty years earlier. While there, she had been diagnosed with Non-Hodgkin's Lymphoma, so I sought her out hoping she could offer me some advice on how to handle what I was about to endure.

To be clear, like snowflakes, no two cancers are the same and no two treatment regimens are the same. But as a human being I knew she could talk to me about what I was feeling. I sent her a DM (Direct Message) on Facebook and asked if I could call her to which she replied yes.

I called her the next day and told her what was going on, what I was feeling, my fears, and as I suspected she was the right person to call. She said she thought something was up based on my Facebook post. Hopefully, if you ever find yourself with a cancer diagnosis you will have someone like her that you can talk to.

I recently became a volunteer "Peer Mentor" through the Cancer Hope Network and I am "coaching" patients through their treatments as well. There are several organizations that offer services like this and if you can't find one, just ask around at the hospital you are being treated at and chances are they will be able to put you in touch with someone who can help you.

Suzanne actually had a friend who lived in my town who also had Multiple Myeloma, so she was very familiar with the chemotherapy regimen they would use and the preparation for and completion of the Stem cell transplant.

I thought this might be a one and done phone call since we hadn't had much contact in the previous twenty years as our careers took on different paths. But she was always there by text or phone if I ever had a question. Occasionally, and this amazed me, she would text me and say things like "Good luck today" or, "You've got this" if she knew the date of an important appointment. Or "Happy Birthday" on the yearly anniversary of my Stem cell transplant, what the doctors and nurses call your "Re-Birthday."

I am so fortunate to have her in my corner and my life, and will never be able to thank her enough for her advice and guidance throughout my journey. The funny thing is she continually thanked me for being there for her while she was going through her cancer journey/fight/battle. I can't recall what I did more than pray for her, and leave her a few motivational notes or cards on her desk, but if it helped, I am glad. I hope you have someone who can be there for you like that.

Another cool thing she did just before I left for the hospital for a two week stay (in isolation) for my Stem cell transplant was send me a care package of ginger lozenges, which helped with the nausea. She also sent me a beautiful blanket with motivational words on it that I brought with me to the hospital and used often. And, I told her I was upset because no Girl Scouts came by my house to sell me my annual three boxes of Trefoil cookies (the best damned cookie ever made!). There in her care package were three boxes of Trefoils. SCORE! I really don't refer to these girls as Girl Scouts, rather I call them my dealers! I have never smoked, never did any illegal drugs, (even when people encouraged me to for the pain in my back), I have never even had a sip of coffee! BUT, you get me near Trefoils and I am 100 percent addicted. It's a shame they only come out in the Spring. I love those cookies.

What also became apparent to me was that many more people than you realize have, or have had, cancer. When we started telling friends, colleagues and family members they would all say something like "Oh my sister had that." Or, "My brother just finished his treatments last month." I was shocked by the number of people who have been affected by this disease, cancer, some of whom I never had a clue were going through this. You probably will be too when you tell people about your situation.

Now it was time to let our inner circle know what was going on with me. We told some people in person and some over the phone and the conversations were always difficult. We told my mother in person along with my sister's. We Gano's are a tough bunch so I don't remember any tears, same with my in-laws. Maybe the shock of it all superseded the tears.

The other shocking part we would later find out was that I now had five (5) compression fractures in my spine. I was getting worse, not better, thus my need for expediting my treatment. I have heard of some people having double digit compression fractures. Five was more than enough for me.

After the holidays, it was time to tell my staff, and my friends which was not easy either. My staff was great and assured me to take care of myself and they would take care of the business, which they did. Again, I only missed a day and a half of work to the chemo treatments in four months, but with my back and constant pain I was working at somewhere between one quarter and one half of my usual self.

There is also a condition you should be aware of if you haven't already experienced it and that is called "chemo brain." Trust me this is real. As you start your chemo treatments you may notice that you are not as sharp mentally as you usually were. Some patients describe it as being in a fog. The thoughts are there, but you just can't speak them. Or a thought will pop into your head and a few seconds later you will forget it. Or you will schedule an appointment or phone call and totally forget to make it. It happens.

The good news is that if you come off the chemo drugs your brain eventually clears the fog. The clearing for me took about six months.

My friends also knew something was wrong, they said they could hear it in my voice. I wasn't my normal self. When they heard I had cancer it came as a shock and I found myself reassuring them everything would be okay rather than the other way around. The only person I told where the reaction bothered me was my best friend, David. We have been friends since we were six years old when he asked me the question, "Is it terminal?" I wasn't ready for that question, not from him. And I hadn't actually thought about that part very much. I hadn't even asked my doctor that question. I replied, "Not if I have anything to do with it." And then I made a bunch of silly jokes that I thought would make him feel better.

Make him feel better? What about me? What would make me feel better? Nothing really. It was my diagnosis and I had to beat it. I'll have more thoughts on this later.

The crazy thing about letting people know was how many of them ran for the hills. No texts, no calls, no check-ins, just silence. Later, some would say, "I didn't want to bother you." But guess what, I wanted to be bothered. I wanted to know that my posse, my friends, my family members were still there. Some were and we would joke around like old times until the conversation circled around to my treatments and we would get serious, but some just left, and in a few cases have never come back. You should prepare yourself for this possibility.

I have to give my in-laws a pass on this. We were dealing with my father-in-law's declining health at this time and about a month after I started my treatments he passed away. I could not imagine what my wife was going through, dealing with me and our all to frequent trips to two different hospitals, and the loss of her father, and taking care of her mother all at the same time, plus working a full-time job. I told her to be there for her mom and I would take care of me. Keep in mind that except for doctor visits and consultations all of my chemo appointments I had to go to myself because of hospital policy during COVID. It was not an easy time for any of us, and I admire my wife for never once complaining.

I remember one night we all went to my in-law's house one morning at two A.M. when my mother-in-law called us and thought the end was near for my father-in-law. Even I went. We stayed up with my mother-in law and father-in-law all night until the sun rose, got them through that night, then I had to leave for a chemo treatment. I actually fell asleep in the treatment chair. I think one nurse thought I was dead, because she kept coming over and touching my arm. I just said, "I'm still here," without opening my eyes.

I will talk later about caring for the caregivers and the sad state of health insurance in this country, but to stay on topic for this chapter, my advice to the patient is when telling family and friends, be honest, answer their questions and encourage them to keep in touch with you. Remember, just as this news was a shock to you, it is also a shock to them. Rather than lamenting the fact that people aren't reaching out to you, force the issue and text them to see how, or what they are doing, it may stimulate a conversation.

Size Matters

Oh, get your mind out of the gutter, this isn't a chapter about that! Just another experience on how cancer can affect you, as it did me.

I wrote earlier about how I needed to have a procedure called a Kyphoplasty done on my back. Actually, I needed five to repair each of the compression fractures in my vertebrae/spine.

As we met with the doctor and talked about the procedure, he said he wanted to perform this before my Stem cell transplant. I had met with another neurosurgeon twice and he refused to do the procedure saying it was too risky on a patient with Multiple Myeloma. When I mentioned this to the doctor who heads up the transplant team, she said "I know a doctor who performs this procedure on Multiple

Myeloma patients all the time."

We set up an appointment with him as he worked in the same hospital and met with him. He reviewed all of my labs, films and did a physical exam and said that I was indeed a candidate for the procedure.

Then he did something amazing and something I had never seen before. He pulled out his cell phone and called the head of the transplant team to inform her I needed the procedure and if he did it that Friday would that allow me enough time to heal before my SCT? To which she replied, yes.

That's the kind of communication I want between the doctor's treating me. Not only communicating as a team on my care, but also not waiting to call at the end of the day or leaving a message in a chart for someone to review at the end of the day, but calling her cell phone and talking it out right in front of me. To say I was impressed is a massive understatement.

The procedure was scheduled for that Friday and went off without any complications. I had to stay overnight, but in the morning, I walked out of the hospital under my own power and with no back brace. I was sore, but I was not in the terrible pain I had been. I could breathe again. If you've ever been in excruciating pain, you know that sometimes you don't take as deep a breath as you normally would.

About a month after the transplant although we still had to be careful of infection, I was told I could kiss my wife. Seriously, prior to this when they said no contact, they meant no contact. When she got a cold during this time she slept in a different bedroom.

Prior to all of this happening I was six feet tall.

23

My wife was five foot three. When we got home, I leaned down to kiss her. I looked at her and she looked at me and I said "do that again." We kissed again and I said "That was too easy." She said "I think you are shorter." We took out a tape measure and I stood against the wall and she measured me and it came out to five foot nine inches. I had lost three inches in height as a result of the compression fractures!

Unfortunately, the Kyphoplasty procedures could only stabilize my spine, not restore my height. I used to enjoy the view at six feet tall, now I was three inches shorter and other than making it easier to kiss my wife I am not a fan of my newfound stature.

However, I am alive and well and living in the land of dreams and despite some stiffness in my back area I am able to do almost everything I did before cancer with some modifications as to how I approach them.

The next side effect I wasn't expecting was that in addition to compressing my spine the loss of height also compressed my insides. My stomach, intestines, liver all vital organs now had to fit in a smaller space which initially was uncomfortable, but I have since gotten used to it. My gut protrudes a little further out despite losing some weight, but compared to the alternative, I'll accept that.

Three inches may not seem like a lot, but I notice that whereas I used to be able to reach things above my head easily, now I am coming up just a little short, but if I find a chair or stepstool, I usually can get it.

Clearly though, size does matter.

"Ain't nothin' gonna come up today..."

If you know me, then you know I am a huge NASCAR fan. I have loved the sport since I was a kid and would see snippets of Richard Petty racing the number forty-three STP car at Daytona on ABC's Wide World of Sports. I have attended many races, met some of the drivers and read many articles and books on the sport. I have met Richard Petty and another favorite driver of mine Mario Andretti on a few occasions and hold both of these gentlemen in very high regard.

1992 would be Richard Petty's last year as a driver so now I was faced with a dilemma, who would I root for? I liked Rusty Wallace, and thought maybe I would root for him. I really liked owner/driver Alan Kulwicki, but unfortunately, he was killed in a plane crash in April of 1993. I had always admired a driver named Davey Allison, a young driver with so much talent, I decided I would start rooting for him. I read everything I could about my new favorite driver and would watch the races on TV as he piloted the number twenty-eight Texaco Havoline Ford around the racetracks every weekend on the NASCAR circuit.

Then in July of 1993 came the tragic news that Davey had been killed in a helicopter crash. He was learning to fly helicopters so he could get to and from the racetracks faster, and get home quicker to his family. My new favorite driver was gone.

But something came of that loss that has stuck with me ever since. A USA Today article referenced a plaque that hung above Davey's office door that read, *"Ain't nothin' gonna come up today that me and the Lord can't handle."*

I have always been a religious person, I even taught CCD at our local Catholic church for five years. My faith has gotten me through many trying times, including cancer. But that one sentence sort of became my mantra in life (you will learn I have many mantras) and I would repeat it to myself almost daily. I noticed that just before my diagnosis I wasn't reciting it as often in the months prior to receiving the news I had cancer. I haven't forgotten to say it once since.

If you are reading this as a cancer patient, your diagnosis may have you questioning your faith and asking "Why me, God?" I will let you sort that out with him and I hope you find the answers you are looking for. But I will say, if you believe, and have faith, don't lose that. There may be times during and after your treatment when your faith will seem to be all you have.

Back to NASCAR for a minute. After Davey Allison died, I started to follow a new driver named

Jeff Gordon. What a talent he was behind the wheel. He had a crew chief named Ray Evernham (another Jersey boy) and Ray too was an exceptional talent at building cars and running the number twenty-four race team. One of the things Ray was also known for being was a great motivator. He had a sign made that he hung in the brand-new race shop at Hendrick Motorsports in big, bold, block letters that read, **"REFUSE TO LOSE!"** Recalling that, it quickly became another mantra for me in my cancer journey. I simply refused to lose to my opponent, in this case Multiple Myeloma.

This next part may sound weird, but I have often talked myself out of being sick. I know what you're saying, *"honey the guy that wrote this book is a nutcase,"* but hear me out. I own my own business so I can't exactly call in sick and lie in bed all day. I have to be there, to make sure the work is getting done, meeting with my customers and making sure my staff has enough work to do.

When I feel a cold coming on, or a headache (I get bad migraines), or a stuffy nose, I will talk to my body and say things like "I'm not sick, I don't have time to be sick, I refuse to be sick." And, the funny thing is that on many occasions within a few hours I will feel better and the next day I won't have any symptoms. I'm not sure if this actually prevents me from getting sick, maybe my subconscious mind takes over and does something to reverse the way I was feeling, but after some time the symptoms aren't there. I have been doing this since high school when I played football. I might get banged up in practice, maybe tweak my knee or hurt my hands, (which are kind of important to a wide receiver) and I would say things to myself like "I'm not hurt, I don't have time for this, we have a game this Saturday, I'm not hurt." The next day, I didn't hurt as much and usually would be able to play in the game. I don't think I ever missed a game in four years. Did my little pep talks have something to do with it? Who knows. But I believe it did.

I don't know how faithful you are, but refusing to lose and reciting the words on Davey Allison's plaque helped get me through every day of my cancer journey.

Is there a phrase or saying or poem that you can use to get you through the trying times? If so, use them, if not you can borrow mine, either way once you receive a diagnosis of cancer, I want you to do one thing ...

REFUSE TO LOSE!

"You're not ready for the storm..."

I am going to talk a lot in this book about motivation and more specifically what motivates me. As I was preparing for a two-week stay in the hospital for my Stem cell transplant, I wanted to have daily reminders to motivate me. I am a history buff so there were many quotes from historical figures that could serve as motivation. Teddy Roosevelt's, *"The Man in the Arena"* comes quickly to mind.

Other times I would pull from quotes from famous sports figures. Pick anything from USA Hockey coach Herb Brooks and I'll be ready to walk through fire. At the end of this book, I have included some of my favorites.

But there was one saying that I saw while trying

to come up with fourteen days of motivation that really stuck with me. I printed it out and took it with me to the hospital. It was a picture of a German Shepherd running toward me and superimposed over the picture was this caption:

"The devil whispered in my ear, you're not strong enough to withstand the storm.

Today I whispered in the Devil's ear, I am the storm!"

BINGO! That one phrase was instantly committed to memory along with others. I now had another mantra, one of many I would use. If I was looking for something to create that "fire in the belly" to make me fight in the hardest times this was going to be it. There are many others and I will share them later, but this was the launch point for me.

I was mad when I was officially diagnosed with cancer. Not at the doctor, but rather at the diagnosis. "I can't have cancer now," I thought. I have too much to do. It was a very inconvenient time for me to get cancer. Now having gone through it I'm not sure there ever is a good time for it.

Going through chemo and reading up on and preparing for the transplant I didn't feel engaged in the process. It was as if I was resigned to just letting the doctors and nurses do what they had to do. Now I was one hundred percent fully engaged. I read more about Multiple Myeloma. I studied the package inserts to my chemo drugs. I read everything I could find about Autologous Stem Cell Transplants. I was informed, and I was ready for the storm.

I was the German Shepherd.

I'm sure many people walk into the hospital for

a chemo treatment or a Stem cell transplant nervous and scared with a fear of the unknown. In my mind I was like "slap that wristband on me, get me upstairs to my room and let's do this." A lot of your success in your treatment and in life, I believe, will have a lot to do with your attitude.

I am reminded of an old motivational speaker from the 1960's named Earl Nightingale. I listened to his cassette tape series (remember those) on my Sony Walkman (remember that? Still have mine) called *"Lead the Field."* On one of the tapes, he talked a lot about attitude.

He equated your attitude with your results this way:

Poor Attitude = Poor Results

Fair Attitude = Fair Results

Good Attitude = Good Results

Great Attitude = Great Results

So, if you or someone you love is currently being treated for cancer how would you rate your/their attitude as it pertains to how they are approaching their treatment? Match their attitude, then compare their results.

As for me, I have always been a person with a positive mental attitude. I look for the good in everything. I am an optimist. I knew I had to be bringing a positive mental attitude and energy to my treatment if I wanted to have a successful outcome. I have zero proof that my attitude helped in my recovery, but I can tell you that I never crawled in bed and allowed myself to feel sorry for my current lot in life, not once.

I would go to chemo at 9:00AM and be sitting at my desk at work by Noon. It would have been much easier for me to take the exit off the highway that led to my house and go home and go to bed on those days, but I just felt I had to show cancer who was boss.

After my transplant I had heard stories and had been warned by the doctors and nurses that I would end up in bed up to eighteen hours a day while I recovered. Sorry cancer, you picked the wrong cowboy this time. I forced myself to wake up at six in the morning, take a shower, eat breakfast and stay awake. It was as if I was reminding my body, "this is how we do things." It was, for lack of a better term, creating muscle memory for my body and my brain. Don't get me wrong in the beginning I was exhausted and often would fall asleep for a few minutes while watching TV. When I awoke, I would walk around my house or yard to keep the blood flowing.

I noticed after about a month and a half I was no longer taking those cat naps during the day, and I was able to stay awake the whole day. And the best part about this time, I was starting to get bored. That was a sign to me that I was getting better.

I am in a support forum group on Facebook for patients with Multiple Myeloma and I read every post. We call ourselves "warriors" because of our battle with cancer. Some posts are encouraging, some are depressing. Many people there will write that they have no energy and lie around all day. Many, like me, have injuries or neuropathy that prevents them from being active. I believe that being active and keeping the blood flowing makes you better.

During the transplant process I had to walk around the hospital floor twenty-three times a day. They had measured it out and that equaled a one-mile distance. Of course, I always tried to complete extra laps. If twenty-three is good, thirty-three is better I thought. So, I would put on my sneakers, grab my I.V. pole, which I affectionately nicknamed "Lucy" and begin my trek around the floor. I think the nurses and other patients got tired of seeing me do my laps, but I didn't care. I was told this would help me get better so I was going to do it.

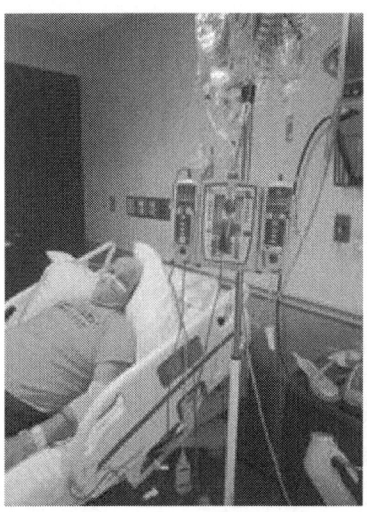

Here I am with "Lucy" my I.V. pole. I literally took her everywhere I went! Look at all those I.V. bags!

It was hard because my back was still sore, but I did it.

More on this later, and throughout this book I will include different quotes I use to get me or keep me motivated. What are some of yours?

The Basement

This chapter deals with a phase you will have to endure if you go through a Stem cell transplant. It is unique to that procedure. The reason I include it as a chapter in this book is that with all cancer treatments there may come a time when you reach the lowest of lows physically and mentally. This chapter describes what happened to me, but you may be able to relate if your treatment knocked the crap out of you too. For the caregiver there isn't much you can do here except monitor the patient, make them comfortable and seek emergency help if needed. It shouldn't be needed, but like a good boy scout, always be prepared.

When you go through a Stem cell transplant there is a phase in your recovery known as "The Basement." This is where all of your blood numbers

I'm Not Done Yet

start to bottom out and slowly you begin to produce (engraft) new healthy cells. The whole transplant process requires a minimum of about two weeks of either in-patient or outpatient treatment.

It is rather anti-climactic compared to the four to six weeks of preparation you go through getting ready for it. There are new medications to take, more lab work, they have to harvest your cells (a procedure known as apheresis), a port has to be inserted and you will have seemingly a million phone calls with your case manager, daily.

A technician comes in with your new cells and reintroduces them through an I.V. line back into your body. It's a lot like receiving a blood transfusion. You almost expect to feel something, but you don't. At least I didn't. Then the technician leaves the room with all her equipment and you wait, and wait, and wait.

A few hours later you feel just as good as you did before they put the cells in you. In fact, you could feel that way for up to five days and then you enter, the basement.

This is where your body starts to accept (hopefully) those new cells that were put back in your body to specifically fight the unhealthy cells and create new healthy ones.

You have no energy. Your brain is struggling to function, you can barely get out of bed. It was only ten feet from my bed to the bathroom and on a few occasions, I didn't make it. All I can say is thank God for Depends™ undergarments. Never, I mean never in a million years did I ever think I would write a sentence like that. But that is how low you get.

Yes, it was humiliating and embarrassing. I

cleaned everything up as best as I could because I did not want to burden the nurses, or anyone else for that matter with having to clean me up, or clean up after me. They all told me that that was their job, but I couldn't do that to them.

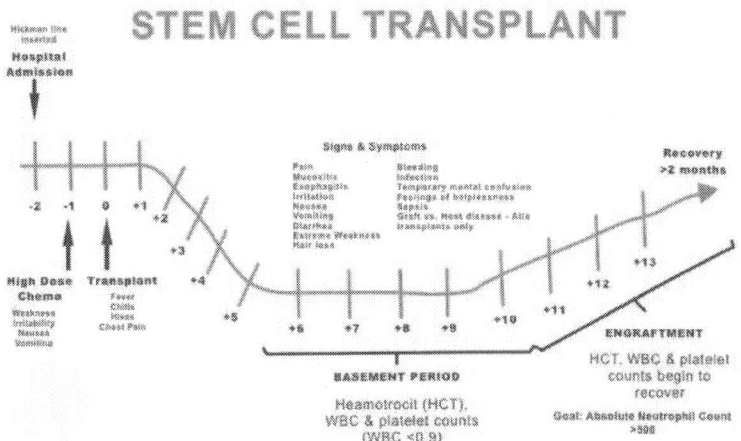

This is a chart describing the timeline of the Stem Cell Transplant process and basement period

I can't recall any time in my life when I was more tired. This was beyond exhaustion and extreme tiredness. I just don't know a word that can best describe it. I would be lying in my bed and start to hallucinate. I imagined that I was visited by friends and family who had been dead for years. At one point I felt as if I was about to die, that this was the end. But then, I mentally told myself NO! I wasn't ready to go. I can remember blinking my eyes, opening them and realizing I was still in my hospital room. With all the energy I could muster, I sat up, took a drink of water, put on my sneakers and started walking. I doubt I was really dying, but that is what my mind thought then, and I wasn't having it.

As the days progressed my blood numbers started to climb and there were certain minimums I had to reach before I could be discharged. I continued my walks around the hallways as best I could all while telling myself, or rather convincing myself this was helping me. I really feel/felt that getting up and moving was helping to circulate my new cells and as such would make me better sooner.

All I knew was I have never been weaker, or more tired, in my life. I struggled to stay awake, to make coherent conversation with my wife, who remember had to drive an hour to visit, so I felt the least I could do was try to stay awake for her. The nurse, Gail, who sat with me during the apheresis procedure told me she came to visit me, but saw I was sleeping and didn't want to bother me. (More on her later).

I tried to stay awake to listen to what the doctors and nurses were telling me about my medications, my progress, etc., but there are about five or six days that were a total blur. Then, on May 31st (my actual birthday in case you wanted to send me a gift, or better yet, Trefoil cookies) I was discharged from the hospital and sent home to finish my recovery.

This was still during the pandemic so I could have no visitors, which in hindsight is probably a good thing as I needed to regain my strength and build up my immune system. Plus, if I was going to be taking a lot of naps, I don't think I would have been very good company.

During this time, I continued to walk, not twenty-three laps around a hospital floor, but in my neighborhood. At first, I started slowly by walking to the end of my street to the stop sign. Don't go getting all excited it is only two houses away from my house, but gradually I increased not only the distance, but the frequency of these walks. Over time I was able to make it around the block, then one lap around a nearby park. They say slow and steady wins the race and I assure you I was not winning any races, but I was making progress and that was a win to me.

Every milestone I achieved whether it was a new distance walked, a reduction in the number of naps, or working four hours in my office on a Saturday were wins to me. I started to notice that every three weeks or so I could sense more strength and more stamina returning to my body. Even now, two years post-transplant there are days when I will do something and say, "I couldn't do that a year ago."

I'll take the small victories, however they come.

Listen to your body

Some of the best advice I received during my cancer journey was from a nurse who told me I had to "listen to my body." When I asked her what she meant she said "your body is going to tell you when it is tired. It's at those times when you have to stop and rest." By rest she went on to say that could mean to just sit in a chair, or it could mean take a nap depending on how tired you are.

In the beginning, shortly after my transplant I understood what she meant. A simple walk around the block could wipe me out for a couple of hours and I would have to sit on the couch and take it easy, or go to bed.

I equated it to me being an iPhone™. I would start the day at one-hundred percent battery. As the day wore on my battery meter, or stamina would start to decrease. By the time dinner rolled around I'd be getting a warning like, low battery and would need to recharge. As I got further along in my recovery and eventually returned to work, I would come home and immediately lie down for at least a half-hour to let my body recover. There were days driving the twelve-mile trip home when I wasn't sure I'd be able to stay awake for the whole drive, but somehow, I made it.

Two years post-transplant there are days when I still need to do this. My naps or rest periods may not need to be as long, but my body appreciates them just the same.

Listening to your body is not just for the patient. The caregiver, the person who is helping the patient has to be mindful of their own well-being as well. And the patient has to respect that. Caregiving of a cancer patient is a 24/7 job. Because even if this person isn't shuttling you to an appointment or somewhere else, they have other tasks they may need to look after. Cooking, cleaning, laundry, dosing meds, whatever the chore, they are there. And even if it doesn't involve a particular task, their brain is constantly thinking about you and what's next. Never take them for granted. And never mistreat them, they are there for you.

They need a break and if you are the patient you have to let them have it. Maybe they want to go out to dinner with their friends, or a movie, or just get away for a little while, let them. Just like you need to recharge your batteries, so do they. The last thing you need or want is a caregiver that stops caring because they just don't have the energy anymore.

It doesn't mean they don't love you or care for you, it just means they need a break. At one point during my recovery my wife's friends arranged for a "girls' weekend" down the shore (you can tell I'm from New Jersey if I say 'down the shore'). I practically begged her to go. She made sure I had enough meals, her mother also only lives just a few miles away, we had plenty of family and friends nearby if I needed anything, so she went.

You could see when she returned from her trip, she had a great time and she couldn't wait to tell me all about it and with such animation in her voice. She needed that break and guess what? I totally survived those two days all by myself. And you probably can too.

When you start to feel a little stronger, don't overdo it. You could make yourself so weak that you become more susceptible to a cold and won't have the strength to fight it off. Additionally, it can take you even longer to recover so in the beginning, pace yourself. Over time you will know how far you can go.

As an example, at the time of this writing for the last six weekends I have been helping my younger son build a deck/platform off his house. One is twelve feet in the air, the other is five, then we have to do the steps and railings. I am two years post-transplant and as little as a year ago, maybe even six months ago I wouldn't have been able to help. But now, I strap on my tool belt, grab my tools and work side by side with him all day on the weekends, and I am loving it.

The best part is, I am not tired or worn out. I'm not even sore. I consider it another milestone in my recovery and it gives me the confidence that I can do even more. (Watch out world, I'm coming for you!) There are certain things I can't and won't be able to do because of my back like golfing because of the torquing motion of the swing, but working on this deck project has shown me that there is probably a lot more that I _can_ do, that before I didn't think I could.

I love passing new milestones and consider myself still recovering even two years later, but man it feels good when I can say I'm almost back to where I was before cancer and in some cases, maybe even better.

Caregivers

In the last chapter I mentioned caregivers, but I want to do a deeper dive on that topic here.

For my type of cancer, Multiple Myeloma, there are several support groups online. I happened across one on Facebook that has been very supportive and best of all informative as I navigated the various stages of treatment. It is called the "Multiple Myeloma Support Group (non-profit)" and I am sure that almost every other form of cancer has some type of support page out there on the web, you just have to search for a while or ask your care provider if they recommend any of them.

I highly suggest that both the patient and the caregiver join some form of a support group whether it is an online forum or a peer-to-peer type through one of the many cancer support organizations. There is something to be said about being able to talk to someone who has already experienced what you are going through and kind of 'walk you through it.'

Although I have already coached three people who were diagnosed with Multiple Myeloma through their treatments, I recently became a Peer-To-Peer mentor through an organization called the Cancer Hope Network. It feels so good to help others and my first patient told me he was so glad he made the call to talk to someone as it has allayed many of his fears toward his treatment. I assured him I would be with him every step of the way and he could call me day or night. I'm not going anywhere, and hopefully I can help him through this.

A word of caution though, you will get to know some of these people on a personal level. You might even call them friends and then one day a family member or friend will write a post that will tear your heart out saying "I am sorry to inform you that my (sister, brother, mom, dad, aunt, uncle, grandmother, grandfather) lost their fight last night." I hate when I read those posts, because as a community we all root for each other, and encourage each other to keep fighting to achieve what we all hope for, a cure or remission.

In these cases, I will say a prayer for them and their loved ones and recall just how lucky I am to still be here and remind myself to never take a minute for granted. It may be one of the reasons I jumped at the chance when I was asked to be a peer mentor.

There is one group of people that I want to talk about that to a certain degree remain in the shadows of a person who has been diagnosed with cancer, and that is their caregiver. This person could be a spouse, partner, relative, friend, maybe they had to pay someone to accompany them because there was no one else closer to help.

Whoever it is, the person with cancer needs to remember that as hard as your diagnosis is on you, it is equally hard on your family, friends and loved ones and especially hard on your caregiver. You have to be mindful that they will be giving up a significant amount of time away from their jobs, or family, to shuttle you to appointments, or sit with you during treatments or visit you during hospital stays. Some might cook meals, clean your house and do the daily tasks that you physically aren't capable of doing as you go through your treatments and as you recover from them later.

Let these people know how much you appreciate them. Tell them you love them if they are a spouse, or family member, or that you appreciate what they are doing, but please don't take the caregivers for granted. It's okay to talk to them about your disease, but every now and then ask them how they are doing and what they are feeling. Maybe they need a break and another person can take care of you for a day, but don't let them suffer because they won't complain to you about what they are feeling. They feel you have enough on your plate, so they keep their concerns and fears to themselves, feeling they have to be strong and brave for you.

There is something else I want you to be mindful of, some chemotherapy drugs can really screw with your brain. You might have been the nicest person in the world before your diagnosis, then the chemo drugs kick in (not all, but some) and suddenly you are a raging lunatic snapping at everyone about anything. I tell people to "find their neutral" in these cases. Let me explain what I mean by that.

There were times during my treatment when one of my drugs, Darzalex would screw with my brain. I had told my wife, and myself, that at any time during treatment if she felt I was being mean or nasty toward her she had to let me know right away. I also reminded myself not to lash out at others. What I told myself and my wife was that I had to find my neutral. Meaning I knew what my good moods felt like and I called that 'my neutral' and I had to remind myself to be that person when I would get upset and not the crazy monster lurking within me. I was actually very good at keeping him at bay. As upset as I might get about something it wasn't my wife's or kid's fault, or my employee's fault it was the medicine so I had to remind myself to get my attitude back to neutral. I could not take my frustrations out on them.

I asked them afterward how I did and they all told me I never once treated them badly. I appreciated them and wanted them to know it. I told them I loved them often, because I wasn't sure how much longer I would be able to tell them that, and I wanted them to know.

Just like the cancer patient needs care and rest so do the caregivers. They stress over everything, your meds, your weight, your eating habits, etc. They may not express it to you but they are constantly worried about you. Please don't make it harder on them by letting the monster within unleash on them.

Depending on who is caring for you, you can send them flowers to thank them. Or maybe buy them a bottle of wine or whiskey. Even a simple thank you card will show them you appreciate their efforts. Don't take them for granted. Have I said that enough times?

I hate when I read on the forum page of my support group that a caregiver is at their wit's end because the person they are caring for, usually a spouse, is so mean to them all the time. I might write a comment of encouragement to them and suggest they mention this to the patient to make them aware of it, because often times you aren't aware of how you are acting or talking to someone when you are on these drugs.

If I know the patient themselves are on the forum board, I might write an occasional post to remind them to find their neutral as well. I hope it helps.

One of the patients I am mentoring told me that he has been mean to his wife a few times. Finally, I asked him, "How are you feeling right now?" he said he was doing well. I asked him if he thought he could take his wife out to dinner and he said yes. I then told him to do it, and make sure she gets dessert too, and at some point in the evening tell her thank you and that you love her. He did and the next time we talked he was beaming about how happy that gesture of taking her out to dinner made her feel so good.

You know how there is a day for everything, like "Taco Tuesday" or "National Chocolate Chip Cookie day?" There is also a National Caregivers Day. It is the third Friday of February every year. Now, go mark your calendars and on that day make sure you do something to show them you appreciate them.

Then imagine for a minute how you would have done all you did without their help.

Trust, but verify

These words were used often by President Ronald Reagan during the nuclear disarmament talks with Russian leader Mikhail Gorbachev back in 1987. Chances are you are not trying to reduce the number of nuclear warheads between both countries, but the phrase "trust, but verify" is still applicable to you during your cancer journey/fight.

Why? Because you are going to get bombarded with information during this time. Information about treatment plans, insurance, nutrition, finances, you name it and somebody will talk to you about it.

If your doctor has told you that you have cancer, is that enough for you? You might want to get a second opinion. When they suggest a treatment regimen, you might want to research if this is the most up to date form of treating your particular cancer.

I have met several people who, once diagnosed, tell me they are traveling all over the country to seek the best treatment. Guess what, sometimes the best treatment is in your own back yard. My wife in her years as a cancer researcher would monitor studies at all the biggest and best cancer centers. You name them, she's been there, MD Anderson, Memorial Sloan Kettering, The Mayo Clinic, The Cleveland Clinic and several top research hospitals and universities along the way.

With her relationships to some of the top cancer doctors and researchers in the country, she probably could have gotten me treated anywhere. The funny thing was after meeting with my doctor's she told me "We don't have to go anywhere, these people are tops in their field."

If she was comfortable with them, then so was I. She did "trust, but verify" all they were saying, and on a few occasions would talk to the actual people who helped develop some of the chemotherapies I would be on. She did her own research and was comfortable with the plan laid out for me.

That was all I needed to hear. Now all I had to focus on was going to the appointments, letting the medicine do its job, and getting better.

I realize as you read this that not everyone is married to a person with thirty-four years of cancer research experience, but the point is simple, you have to advocate for yourself. If you can't do it, then your caregiver must. Make sure you have all of the questions answered and have no doubts or reservations about your care.

If something doesn't make sense, question it. If

a doctor won't take the time to answer all of your questions, find a new doctor. This is literally your life we are talking about here. Think back to when you were first diagnosed. At first there was the shock and fear that we all feel when we hear those words, "you have cancer." The fear of the unknown I call it. But those feelings were probably replaced with hundreds if not thousands of questions. Write them down and bring them with you to your next appointment and get them answered. Be like the investigative reporters you see on the TV news. Keep digging for answers until you are satisfied.

If a doctor or Nurse Practitioner is dismissive or won't take the time to answer your questions, get rid of him or her. Find someone who will.

That is also a warning shot to all doctors and nurses who may be reading this. We have questions, you have the answers, we need them. Take the time before, during and after diagnosis to put the patient at ease.

I am a sports guy. I played sports, I coached sports so a lot of my analogies revolve around sports. I joked with my doctor and nurse practitioner and eventually with anyone responsible for my care, "welcome to the team" when I first met them. What I meant was that anybody who was going to be treating me from any department had to work together and treat the "whole" me and not just their area of expertise.

Obviously, there was Oncology involved, but because of my back issues and coming off surgery just three weeks prior to my transplant we also had to include Neurosurgery. Everybody that had a hand in my care had to know what everyone else was doing. I insisted on it. I questioned if the oncologist was recommending a drug how would it interact with something the neurosurgeon might prescribe or suggest, or the transplant team. Or if it would have an impact on any medication I was taking prior to my diagnosis. Because we were in this game together. This was my team, and we weren't about to lose this game. At one appointment my doctor entered the room and said "hi, coach." He got it.

Eventually, after I went through all the treatments and was declared in remission, I changed that message from "welcome to the team," to "welcome to the family." I love these people for what they did for me. They gave me a second chance and I am going to take it, and make the best of it, every day.

During our initial meetings after they laid out the treatment plans for me, they would actually encourage me to seek a second opinion either in network, or out of network which gave me the confidence that they believed in their plan. If they believed, and my wife believed, then so did I.

But first I had to trust, but verify.

Cancer does not define me

The last thing I wanted from cancer was for that to be what people remembered me for.

I get upset when I read an obituary in the newspaper that says someone "lost their battle" with cancer. What else did they do? What did they do for a living, or career? What were their interests, hobbies, etc.? But for so many people the first three sentences will give their name, where they lived, when they died and their cause of death, cancer. I remember reading about one gentleman who held over one hundred patents. But that was nearly an afterthought at the end of his obituary.

When people meet me for the first time, they are shocked to hear I once had cancer if it comes up in conversation at all. Trust me, I don't bring it up, usually someone else will make mention of it. Then I'll have to explain all I went through. I don't want my disease to define who I am. And I certainly don't want anybody's pity. I have done a lot in my life from my career(s), to my volunteer work, to employing people, to being a published author, a podcast host, a coach, an announcer and so much more. That is what I want to be remembered for, not that I died of cancer, or that I even had it. I hope I'll be remembered for being a good husband, father, son, uncle, cousin (not necessarily in that order Mom) and not just some guy who had cancer.

I have often said "I won't let cancer kill me." I might step off a curb and get hit by a bus, but I won't let cancer be my demise.

During my treatments, if I was going to a meeting or a public event, I could see the stares and hear the whispers of people. The same people I had had meetings with before, only now, I had cancer. And they knew it, and they were telling others.

Funny how while volunteering on some of these committees I still got more done than my healthy counterparts, but that is probably a subject for another book. I like to be involved, and get involved and contribute to an organization's success, not just sit on the sidelines and take the credit for someone else's work.

A funny side note is that now, two years after being declared in remission when people see me for the first time, they'll say something like "you look great." I tease them and say, "you know prior to cancer you never said that about me." One guy, an actual funeral director said it differently when he said "you look alive." I said, "sorry to disappoint you." A little gallows humor among friends. I think they mean they are happy to see me and that I look healthy. I'm not sure how they thought I would look, but I appreciate the compliments all the same.

There was one troubling yet funny story I will share with you that shows how quickly things can get out of hand if you let them. PS, don't let them.

As I mentioned, I own my own business, an awards and promotional products company along with a sign shop. I hadn't told my customers, nor was I planning to, what I was going through. Then one day a longtime customer of mine whom I consider a friend called me up and said, "Hey, I'm sorry to hear you have to close the business because you have cancer."

I said, "I'm not closing the business. Where did you hear that?"

He said, "You know, people were talking and someone said you weren't doing well and had to close the business."

"Well tell them I'm not closing the business," I instructed him.

A few weeks passed and he called again. "Hey, I'm sorry to hear you have to sell the business because you have cancer."

I said, "I'm not selling the business. Where did you hear that?"

He said, "You know, people were talking and someone said you weren't doing well and had to sell the business."

"Well tell them the business is not for sale." I instructed him.

A few more weeks passed and this same friend called me and was chuckling a little as he started talking. I said, "What's up?"

He said, "I'm sorry to hear you have to close the business because you died."

I hate the rumor mill. And this last one cost me a lot of time, energy and yes, money. I had to issue press releases, make posts on social media, call key customers to assure them I was not dead, sit for interviews with newspapers who wanted to report the story. All because some numbskull, who didn't have the right, or any correct information decided to run his or her mouth off.

The most important lesson out of all this is that I had to control the messaging. I couldn't let the rumor mill run wild or I would have been out of business within six months. This also applied to family members and friends as well. I had to stay in front of the messaging so I would often group text people and update them on my progress and how far along I was on my treatment regimen. This way everyone got the same message at the same time. I could not let the rumor mill run the message, or people would be wondering if I would be wearing my blue suit or gray suit at my funeral. To be honest I don't care which suit I wear, just pick out one of my Jerry Garcia ties. I love those.

I hope my obituary doesn't even mention that I ever had cancer. I hope during my lifetime that I accomplish so much that the newspapers write about that, and there won't be any room for any mention of cancer. It simply does not define me, or who I am. In my mind, I had it, got treated for it, beat it for now and I am moving on. Kind of like a long, bad cold. A very simple view, but hopefully you get my drift, cancer does not define who I am.

Ultimately, the business survived. I survived, but it underscored the need for me and you to control our own narrative. That is why you have to make sure key people, friends, family, bosses, co-workers, etc., know what's going on. Don't let the rumor mill take control of your story.

Or you might end up dead . . . like me!

Ringing the Bell

There are many instances where people reference bells. In the movie *"It's a Wonderful Life"* the angel Clarence tells George Bailey played by Jimmy Stewart that "every time a bell rings, an angel gets its wings." In boxing, the sound of the bell means the end of a round.

In the context of Navy SEAL training, ringing the bell signifies a trainee's voluntary withdrawal (or quitting) from the program. Navy SEAL training, also known as BUD/S (Basic Underwater Demolition/SEAL training), is notoriously grueling and demanding both physically and mentally. The bell itself is typically located near the training area and is rung by trainees who have decided they can no longer continue with the rigorous demands of the program.

Conversely, in the context of someone who is in

the process of undergoing treatment for cancer, ringing the bell is a sign of achieving a meaningful milestone in their journey through cancer treatment, particularly in the context of completing a course of chemotherapy or radiation therapy. Like SEAL training, cancer treatment is notoriously grueling and demanding both physically and mentally. The tradition of the "bell ringing ceremony" varies across different hospitals and treatment centers, but its significance is generally universal.

For the patient who has just completed treatment it provides a sense of hope and achievement after enduring that line of treatment. For the other patients going through treatment hearing someone ring the bell offers hope and inspiration that they too will one day achieve that milestone. It reminds them that others have travelled the same path they are now on and won their battle for the moment. It gives them hope.

The bell ringing ceremony is often a moment of acknowledgment and celebration not only for the patient, but also for their healthcare team, family, and friends who have supported them along the way. It honors the collective effort and commitment to fighting cancer. To be clear, it is a collective effort.

Beyond celebration, ringing the bell can also represent a sense of closure for the patient as they move from active treatment to the next phase of their cancer journey, whether it's ongoing monitoring, recovery, or transitioning back to everyday life.

Overall, the act of ringing the bell for a cancer patient is deeply significant, symbolizing not just the end of treatment but also a powerful affirmation of hope, resilience, and the determination to overcome cancer. It marks a moment of triumph and serves as a beacon of encouragement for others facing similar challenges.

So, what was it like when I got to ring the bell?

I don't know.

I never got that opportunity. I was scheduled for six cycles of chemotherapy before I was scheduled to begin the preparation for my Stem cell transplant. Every week I would go for my chemo session(s) and as I walked out at the end I would have to pass the bell in the hallway. I would look at it and long for the day when I could grab that rope and triumphantly ring the hell out of that bell.

After the fourth cycle, I was told my blood numbers had gotten into a satisfactory range (actually they said I had made "remarkable progress") where I could stop the chemo and begin the next phase, prepping for the Stem cell transplant. This was told to me in my doctor's office on the second floor of the hospital. The bell was on the third floor. Just one floor separated me from the moment I had been thinking about for twelve weeks. I thought for a moment about going upstairs and ringing the bell in celebration, but there was a new phase to prepare for. Although the chemo phase was over, the hard work was just beginning, the bell would have to wait.

During a follow up visit with my doctor many months later I heard someone ring the bell and I was happy for them. I could picture the scene with the individual surrounded by nurses and doctors and family. I was truly happy for them. As I drove home a tear formed in my eye as I realized I hadn't gotten to experience that feeling with my care team, or my wife. Hopefully not, but maybe one day I will have that chance if my cancer ever recurs.

Most importantly for cancer patients is that unlike the Navy SEALS, we can never quit, failure is not an option. So, to all my fellow cancer patients when you get the chance, ring that bell.

An Attitude of Gratitude

I've already written about your need to show your gratitude to your caregiver, but if you want to make your treatment a little easier, show the same gratitude to your doctors and nurses. I'll take it one step further, show it to anyone you come in contact with who in some way plays a role in your care. This includes any technicians, orderlies, even the people that mop your floors and clean the dirty linen bins and wastebaskets in your hospital room.

Have "an attitude of gratitude" towards these people. We all think of the doctors and the nurses who are caring for us, but everybody contributes to our care.

How did I do it. Simple, and it only cost me a few bucks. I bought a two-pound bag of LifeSavers™

candies and put them in a cup on a counter in my room. Anybody who walked in that room I told them I had some candies in the cup on the counter. They happily helped themselves to the candies as a treat for themselves during the day.

Now let's be clear I wasn't sharing my Girl Scout cookies, but they could have some candy. Nobody touches my Girl Scout cookies!

And a funny thing happened along the way. Everybody started visiting me a little more frequently. My wastebasket was always empty, I had all the supplies I needed in the bathroom, they brought me extra blankets. It was their way of saying thanks to me for showing my appreciation to them.

And I didn't just rely on the candy. Remember I was in their care for two weeks, so I started talking to them and getting to know them and they in turn got to know me. They asked about my family, my Grandkids, they asked to see pictures. They loved when I showed them pictures of my antique car, a 1948 Plymouth Special Deluxe (Go ahead, Google it, you know you want to).

I took it a step further and tried to learn all of their names as well. There is something unique about greeting someone by their first name, rather than just a hello. And I took just as much pleasure in learning about them and their families. I actually started to miss our daily visits when I was discharged from the hospital.

One lab tech was Polish so every morning when she entered the room to take my blood I would say, "Dzień dobry" (pronounced Jeen Do-bray) which means Good Morning. It's the only word I know in Polish other than Kielbasa and Pierogies (one of my favorite meals), but it created a connection between her and I.

One nurse came in my room one day and said "You're holding out on me." I asked, "How so?" She said "I Googled you. You didn't tell me you were an author, now I'm treating a celebrity." I replied, "I may be a published author, but I assure you I am no celebrity." We talked about writing and she politely asked for a copy of my book, *"The Player"* which I had my wife bring to the hospital the next day for her.

Who knows if they'll ever think of that guy from room 8008 that asked them all those questions, but I assure you, a couple of years removed from my transplant, I still think of them.

And I treated everyone like this from the techs in the lab who took my blood, to the people who would deliver my food, or what appeared to be food every day. (We really have to work on institutional cuisine).

I noticed listening to other rooms that they wouldn't even so much as say hello when these people entered their rooms. Little did they know that if you treated them nice, they might even bring you an extra Jell-O™ (hint, hint).

Okay this is starting to sound like a prison novel and I don't want to make that comparison. The point is, help make your stay as comfortable as possible by getting to know these people and they will do what they can to help you.

To be clear it can be hard depending on the drugs you are on which can alter your mood. Just be nice.

I was in the hospital on my actual birthday and the nurses came in with a cupcake and balloons and signs they had made. Maybe they do this for every patient on their birthday, but they sang Happy

Birthday to me, and took great joy in trying to make my day special. I really appreciated that and even told them so.

Doctors came around on rounds and I remember one nurse was with them and she sort of did a tap dance and screamed "woo-hoo" when she realized it was my birthday. Everybody laughed and congratulated me.

The lead doctor looking to restore order said, "Okay, I'd like to review your labs."

I said, "Not until you dance and scream woo-hoo, like she did." And he actually did it! We all had a good laugh together before reviewing my labs.

One doctor from those rounds came into my room later and said she had never seen the lead doctor act that way and thanked me for showing him it was okay to act that way in front of a patient. Otherwise, he was always a by the book kind of doctor. Who knows if he has ever danced for another patient, but I do know one thing, he did for me!

Hair Loss

This is a tough chapter to write about and I am sure it will be a tough one to read about and experience. But, like I said earlier you're getting the good, the bad and the ugly with this book.

Hair loss. It is inevitable for most cancer patients. Oddly, when my grandfather was being treated for cancer in the 1970's he never lost his hair. That is usually the exception with most chemo drugs today.

When I was a kid, my mother would usually make my sisters and I accompany her on her errands which included occasional trips to the beauty parlor. I would sit in a chair and watch the ladies under the hair dryers reading Cosmopolitan magazine or talking, and just bide my time until we could go home.

65

Seemingly on every trip to the beauty parlor some woman would make a comment about my hair and tell me what beautiful hair I had. In my early teens in the 1970's my hair was a little longer and a lot curlier and browner than it is now. Some of these women would even get out of their chair to touch my hair (a little creepy by today's standards).

Eventually we would finally go home and I wouldn't have to deal with this for a few more weeks until my mother's next appointment.

When I was prepping for my Stem cell harvest, my wife and I decided to get a room in a hotel near the hospital for a few days as we lived an hour away from the hospital and the daily commute was wearing us out. A new drug was administered that they told me could make my hair fall out. I had tried to imagine what I would look like bald, but never could.

Please don't think I am vain with this next sentence. I'm an okay looking guy, but I don't spend a lot of time on my appearance. I only look in the mirror once a day and that is because it hangs above my sink in the bathroom. I brush my teeth and my hair once in the morning and that is it as far as my beauty regimen goes for rest of the day. (I do brush my teeth at night).

One night in the hotel I got up around two-fifteen in the morning as I had to go to the bathroom. I remember scratching my head above my temple and when I pulled my hand away, I saw a clump of hair in my fingers. I threw out the hair and pulled at the spot again and sure enough more hair was now in my hand.

It was happening.

My hair was beginning to fall out, and so did my tears. I wept and I don't know why. I knew this was a possibility, if not a probability. Every doctor and nurse said it would happen, but when it actually did, I got emotional. I got myself to stop crying then went back to bed. I just laid there in the darkness wondering what I would look like bald and trying to accept the fact that I was now entering a new phase in my cancer journey. When we woke up in the morning, I told my wife what happened during the night.

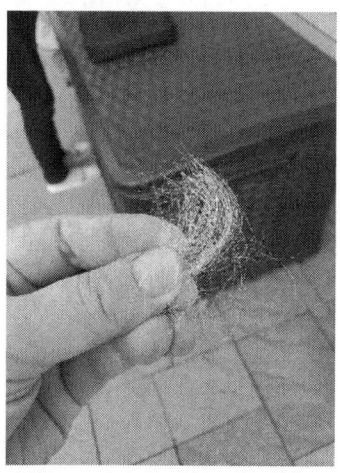

And so it begins, the first clumps of hair begin to fall out

This was a new experience for her because for her entire career in cancer research patients were just numbers on a page to protect their privacy. She never knew a patient's name or met them, so if a report came in that a patient had a serious adverse event to a drug she was studying, it was just patient number 018476, not Mrs. Marion Smith of Paducah, Iowa having the reaction.

Now, she was seeing first-hand what a cancer patient was going through. I think she appreciated the patient side of the research more after that.

I knew this upset her, but she never showed it. She just said it was okay and we would deal with it.

When we got home a couple days later, I told her to get the clippers and shave my head. I wasn't going to wait for it all to fall out in clumps I would be proactive and do it myself. She cut my hair to within an eighth of an inch, peach fuzz length, and the rest thinned out considerably, but never completely fell out.

Even though I knew we had shaved my head it was still a shock the next morning to see the guy staring back at me in the mirror. It took a few days, but eventually I got used to it. I had read on the forum board that it would grow back and some said it would come in darker and curlier. Mine grew back straight and the same gray it had been before it started falling out.

The hard part was explaining to my grandchildren who were ages three and one at the time why Pop Pop didn't have any hair. I didn't want to scare them about medicine or doctors, so I simply told them I cut it off. I let them rub my head and we turned it into a game called "fuzzy wuzzy." They would rub my head and yell out "fuzzy wuzzy, fuzzy wuzzy!" I didn't mind and at least they weren't afraid of my new look.

The good news is my hair eventually grew back. My rationalization during this one-year period was 'look how much money I'm saving by not getting a haircut every four weeks.' It was strange looking in the drawer in the vanity cabinet every day and seeing my hair brush just sitting there as if to say "pick me, pick me." But I didn't need it for about eight months. This really sped up my prep time in the morning too.

If you are facing hair loss, I recommend you not wait. When it starts falling out, get rid of it. Prepare yourself emotionally, but it is better to me than suffering through the clumping that happens to some patients. I saw a documentary on tennis legend Chris Evert recently where she started wearing wigs during her most recent bout with cancer. Now, they even make wigs sewn into baseball caps, and she looked great. You could not tell any of them were wigs.

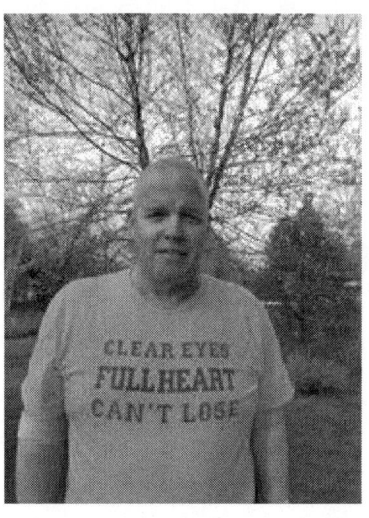

Me after we shaved my head. It was definitely a different look. Also, this is the tee shirt I had made up with my mantra, "Clear Eyes. Full Heart. Can't Lose."

I know it will be more difficult for some, particularly women, as if the hair loss makes your cancer real, but trust me once it's gone you can deal with it better, rather than watching it slowly fall out.

And besides, you'll save all that money by not having to go get your hair cut!

No Pain, No Gain

Show of hands, how many people have ever heard that saying, or have even said that saying? Okay put your hands down your reading a book, not playing Simon says.

If you've ever played sports or trained for an event like a marathon or 5K or 10K, something requiring physical preparation you might have heard that phrase.

Some guy in the gym might yell over to you, *"hey buddy, no pain, no gain!"*

Well, here is the deal, they've probably never had to deal with a cancer diagnosis. Many of the very drugs and treatments that we are given as patients to 'heal us', actually hurt us physically first.

One of the steps in preparing for my Stem cell transplant required me to give myself twice daily injections of a drug called Neupogen. This drug is used to help the body make white blood cells after receiving cancer medications. I had to do this for five days, each day I was going to be hooked up to the apheresis machine, one shot in the morning and one at night.

Some people can collect enough cells in one day, but not me. No, it took me five days to collect twelve million cells. Thus, all the shots. On the fourth and fifth day realizing I still wasn't producing enough cells they doubled the dose.

They prep you in advance by telling you to take Claritin™ to offset the pain that invariably comes with taking the drug. They didn't advise what would happen if they doubled the dosage. By the fifth night I was in agony. I normally have a very high tolerance for pain. I have played sports with broken bones and never complained about pain. But this was unlike anything I have ever experienced in my life.

I used to work in a delicatessen and butcher shop in high school. I would watch the butcher, Mr. Vaughn, take a cleaver and split a chicken in half with one whack of the blade. That is what I felt was happening to me in my hip area. I felt like I was being split apart. To be honest every bone in my body ached as the medication was hyper forcing cell production.

We called the nurse's line at the hospital and there was no answer so we left a message. We called my original hospital and there was no answer there either. Finally, at nine o'clock that night I asked my wife to take me to the hospital where they could either give me something for the pain, or shoot me, I really didn't care which at this point, just make the pain stop.

We got in the car and just as she was about to put the car in drive to leave, my phone rang. We told the nurse what was going on and she was concerned and asked what pain medications we had in the house. The only thing I could think of was Oxycodone which I had been prescribed but did not use for my knee replacement surgery. She told me to take two pills every three hours, basically doubling the normal dosage and to call if the pain did not subside.

Finally, at around four in the morning I fell asleep or passed out, I'm not sure which. That was the worst night of my life pain wise, and I wouldn't wish that on anyone.

Other drugs and treatments like radiation and chemo can cause pain. Do not allow yourself to suffer. Consult with your physician to see if there is something you can do to alleviate it.

Here is a note of caution though that was shared with me by a nurse when I told her that story. When they say take Claritin™ or any drug such as Tylenol™ they are referring to the name brand and dosage and not a generic or proprietary drug store brand, but the real thing.

So, I had the pain, but not sure I got the gain. Unless you want to say the transplant was successful and I am still in remission.

In that case all I can say is no pain, no gain.

The Gift

A few years ago, I interviewed a couple on my radio show about their family business. It was a great interview if I do say so myself, and it seemed like it was just a conversation among friends rather than an interview to learn about their business. We developed a friendship from this time and kept in touch.

Several years passed and now the woman, Michaela, wanted to interview me on her podcast. As we had conversations leading up to the interview, she mentioned to me that her husband had recently been diagnosed with MS, Multiple Sclerosis. She assured me that he was doing fine now, but that disease can become debilitating when it becomes active.

Talking about him and my cancer diagnosis she said something very interesting, "I hope you both realize what a gift you've been given with your illnesses."

I was like, "I don't think too many people would consider cancer or MS a gift."

She clarified by saying, "you two get to look at life through a different lens now. Everything has changed for you. You are probably thinking of things, like your mortality, which you never gave a second thought to before."

She was right. One-hundred percent right. I had never thought about that, at least not as much as I was now. I've had a few health scares in my life before, and working on a rescue squad I've had a few 'my life passed before my eye's moments', but once I survived those episodes it was back to business as usual. I never thought about my own mortality, that is until a doctor told me I had cancer.

The funny thing to me is that thinking about it, I wasn't focused on me. I thought about my wife, my kids, their kids. I wanted to be around for my younger son's wedding, I wanted to watch them flourish in their careers. I wanted to see their children grow and go to their tee-ball games and dance recitals.

I didn't want to be the empty chair that exists in so many households where a loved one used to sit, but is no longer there.

Suddenly her words about "the gift" I had received was starting to come into clearer focus. Within days I started to notice a change in myself. Little things that used to bother me didn't anymore. I also wasn't getting angry at things if they weren't done a certain way. I tried to learn new things every day, about the world around me and myself.

I started to pay attention more to nature and the simplest things in life like a bird flying or that crazy little groundhog that lives under my shed searching for food. I wasn't just paying attention to it. I was getting absorbed into it. Everything was beautiful in some way if I would allow myself the time to appreciate it.

I no longer got mad at the idiot driver that cut me off on the highway. He obviously had somewhere more important to go to than I did. I calmed down. As I did, I noticed all the people around me who had never received the gift, who were uptight, always in a hurry, seemingly never satisfied with anything in life and I laughed.

Not cancer, but I wish I was given this gift so many years earlier, because I was that uptight, always in a hurry, never satisfied guy. I just appreciate the little things more now.

I appreciate when an employee makes an extra effort to get something done without being asked. Or if my one son calls and invites my wife and I to breakfast. Or spending time with my other son, his wife and the grandkids, oh and my Granddog too, (sorry Sidney. I love that pup.)

I find I don't get upset with my vendors if they screw up and I am more inclined now to be looking for a solution to the problem rather than lamenting the original problem.

I'm not sure about her, but I really enjoy just being around my wife. It used to bother me when she would tell me stories about what was going on at work or elsewhere and now, I can't get enough. I like those stories and the characters in them, whereas before to me it was just work drama.

If you are dealing with a diagnosis of cancer, I know you have a lot to process. Definitely more than the average human, but at some point, I want you to think about what my friend said about "the gift" we have all received, and see if it doesn't change the lens that you look at life through.

The Little Gray Cloud

I'm going to tell you a story now that may or may not apply to you now, but might someday. It also doesn't matter whether you are the patient, or the caregiver.

When I was initially diagnosed and through the first six months of treatments it felt like I jumped on a treadmill with no off button running at full speed. There were doctor appointments, lab appointments, consultations, second opinions, it got to the point where I felt everyone else was running my calendar and all I was doing was showing up at the prescribed date and time.

Four months of weekly chemotherapy treatments, followed by a month of preparation for the Stem cell transplant, followed by five Kyphoplasty procedures to fix my back, followed by the actual transplant and then finally after two weeks in isolation I was sent home (on my actual birthday) to recover. Still more isolation awaited me until my blood numbers and immune system recovered.

Throughout all of this the country was still in the throes of the COVID-19 pandemic so I had to be extra careful, as did my wife of coming in contact with someone who was exposed to the disease. My immune system had been wiped out and was slowly being built back up. A simple cold could have landed me back in the hospital, let alone if I contracted COVID.

At the one-hundred-day post-transplant mark we met with the doctor who headed up the transplant team and she reviewed my labs with us. At the end of our review, she declared that I was in "complete stringent remission." This was music to my ears. It was now ten months since I had been officially diagnosed and begun treatment, and to hear those words brought us much joy.

I asked her what the next steps were knowing that I could be facing a second or "tandem" transplant in a few months, or a lifetime on maintenance chemotherapy drugs, but she said no, I wouldn't need either. She described my situation as this, "We have enough of your cells to do two more transplants in cold storage. Your numbers look great so I don't want to put you on a drug regimen that might lead me to be treating you for another cancer in five years. We have five drug cocktails we can use with you now if your cancer recurs so I want to leave all of these things in reserve, sort of tools in your toolbox, in case we need them."

My next steps would be to come back every three months for the next two years for lab work and follow up appointments. At these appointments I would also be receiving every vaccination I got when I was a baby because the chemo and transplant would most likely have wiped out the originals.

We left that appointment and were almost giddy knowing I didn't have to do a second transplant or be on any maintenance drugs. To say I am a lucky man is an understatement to say the least.

I was pretty much back at work full-time in September of 2021 unless I got tired in the afternoon and then I would leave a little early. I noticed that cancer was no longer all-consuming and front of mind with me anymore. I could go days without thinking about all that I had been through.

The funny thing to me is that as I went through it. I either didn't think about how hard it was, or didn't know it was hard. I just woke up every day with a "what do I have to do today" attitude when it came to my treatments. It wasn't until one of my doctor's sat me down and explained what I went through and what my body endured that I began to understand the seriousness of it all. I guess maybe I was a lot like Dopey from Snow White, I just kind of whistled while I worked at getting better.

Over time though I noticed something, at any given moment, I would be reminded of my cancer or the transplant process. It could be a sound, a food, (for the longest time I couldn't look at scrambled eggs), a TV show, it didn't matter, something would trigger a memory. It was what I came to call "my little gray cloud." It was as if I was walking around on a beautiful day with a blue sky and no matter where I went this little gray cloud followed me around. Sometimes the cloud would grow larger and more imposing meaning I was becoming all-consumed with memories and fears of cancer. Other times, I felt like I was a strong breeze and would just push the cloud out of sight.

I have mentioned this to other people who have had cancer and they describe having similar feelings. One person said "it's like our own form of PTSD (Post-Traumatic Stress Disorder)." And I believe she was right. It wasn't crippling like you hear about with people returning from overseas in the military, but it would cause you to pause until the moment passed. Sometimes it would pass quickly and other times it might be a few hours, or even days.

I was interviewed on a podcast recently and the host asked me "as long as I've known you, you are the most positive person I have ever met. Do you ever get sad?"

To which I replied, "No." I simply don't allow myself to get sad and dwell on things that might ordinarily bring me down. Don't get me wrong if someone dies, I am upset by this news, we all would be. It is the little things that happen to you that I don't allow to bring me down. I will acknowledge the feeling, but I quickly move on, because I like being happy more than I do sad. I am not in denial, I am not ignoring what normally would or should make a person sad, I simply choose to not let it consume me and be ever-present in my day.

I have been around these people, some have worked for me and if you thought I had a little gray cloud following me around, they were living inside the cloud, and it was always raining. You probably have a friend or two that are like this, nothing is ever right with them, they are always complaining about their situation in life. That is not me. If something is wrong in my life, I fix it. Head on. I don't ignore it. I don't wish it away. I don't hope it will take care of itself. I take care of it. And then I move on.

If you think about how your body feels when you are constantly sad you will probably notice that everything hurts a little more, you're tired more, you have less energy, you delay doing things around the house, you become disengaged.

Now imagine that is how you decided to approach your cancer treatments. I don't know if there are any scientific studies about how your attitude affects your ability to heal, but from my experience I'll take a positive approach to a negative one every day of the week.

If you find that you are more of a negative person, I would challenge you to change your mindset. Look for and find the positive in everything. To steal a line from Randy Pausch's book *"The Last Lecture"* which I highly recommend you read, ask yourself "Are you an Eeyore or a Tigger?" based on the characters in the Winnie the Pooh books.

Me? I'm a "T-I-Double Guh–er" Tigger, every day of the week.

I simply don't know how, nor would I want to be, negative as I approach life, or cancer. Try it for twenty-one days, the time I am told it takes to create a new habit and see if you don't notice a change in yourself.

Survivor vs. *Thriver*

I recently spoke before a business networking group and as the host of the meeting introduced me in addition to reciting my bio information and professional accomplishments said "and, Jim is also a cancer survivor." Did I previously say that cancer wouldn't define me? I thought so. Now I had to get these people to forget what they just heard and focus on the message I was originally brought in to deliver, which in this case was marketing their business. I didn't want the audience feeling sorry for me or looking at me differently just because I had cancer. I started my presentation a little differently this time.

I said, "I was introduced as a cancer survivor and that has absolutely nothing to do with what we are talking about here, marketing your business. It is also a misstatement of the truth. I don't look at myself as a cancer "survivor," rather I think of myself as a cancer "thriver."

Now I had their attention, most people don't use the word thriver to discuss how they fought their cancer, they do use the word survivor and quite proudly I might add, that they survived cancer. And they can and should. But then what? Is that it? You survived cancer, I absolutely applaud you for it, but now there is hopefully a whole lot of living left to do. How will you live it? Are there things you had to put on hold because of your cancer, maybe a trip to Europe, learning a new language, learning to paint, singing in a coffee house on open mic night? What did you have to hit the pause button on in your life because of your diagnosis that if you could you would like to do?

Do it now.

You almost lost that chance once, don't go for two. I have always been the type of person who takes advantage of almost every opportunity that comes my way. If I am invited somewhere I try to go. If someone invites me to do something I've never done before, sign me up (except parachuting out of an airplane, there ain't no reason to jump out of a perfectly good aircraft). But you get my drift. And that has only gotten more intense since I did "survive" cancer.

There are times when my wife and I are both tired and friends may call to invite us out to dinner. Initially, my wife and I both might want to say no, but that thriver mentality makes me say yes. And the funny thing is while we could have stayed home and done nothing, we always have a good time with our friends. We have travelled with them, taken vacations with them, taken day trips with them, gone to dinner with them and we always have a good time.

Someone once asked me how do I get it all done and why do I do it? And I said, "I make the time for it. When I am 80 years old and sitting in the rocking chair on the front porch of the nursing home, I don't want to look back and say, I should have gone on that trip to Europe, or I should have gone to that dinner party where that celebrity showed up. Or I should have taken that job offer." I don't want there to be any regrets in my life and up until this point I can honestly say there aren't many, if any at all.

The point here is this, very few of us ever think about the fact that we only have a finite amount of time on this earth. We put things off for so long until one day we look around and realize there isn't enough time left.

If anything made me realize that, it was cancer, and I am thankful for it. It is so easy to put things off. Now, especially now, when I am asked if I want to do something I say yes, because I don't know if I'll ever have the opportunity again.

Yes, cancer sucks. Let's get that out of the way first, but life doesn't suck, so how do you want to live it, as a survivor, or as a thriver?

I have said in previous chapters that I have been told my cancer will come back at some point (hopefully a long time from now). So why wouldn't I take advantage of every opportunity now, while I can? Nothing in this life is guaranteed. Nowhere have you been given a piece of paper that says "you will live until you are 95." So, you better start living today. Not just living, but thriving.

Since my diagnosis I appreciate everything and everybody so much more. I notice things more that I never used to pay any attention to. I might see a plane flying in the sky leaving a contrail behind it and wonder where are those people going? Or I might see a small animal or bird and watch all of its mannerisms as it scavenges for food.

I definitely look forward to, and love to spend more time with my Grandchildren and see the world through their eyes and answer their many questions. My five-year-old grandson is like my best friend, and I love spending any time with him either in person or on a video call. As a result of the five broken vertebrae in my back and the Kyphoplasty procedure to correct and stabilize it, I'm not as flexible as I used to be, but when my grandkids ask me to get on the floor and play with them, or give them a shoulder ride or a pony ride, I am right there with them saying "hop on."

My wife will say something like "Jim, your back," and I'll say "so what, we're having fun." Usually when we get back home or to a motel room I'll lie down for a while and take some Advil then get ready for the next day. I definitely don't want my grandkids to remember me as the old man who just sat in the chair and watched them play. My hope is they will have memories of me that they will carry with them forever.

That is what I am doing when I spend time with them, making memories. My Grandson and I have a very special bond and I know when the time comes that I am not around he will miss me. He may miss my physical presence, but just like I did with his father I have been teaching him lessons that he will carry with him his whole life. I want him to believe that I will always be with him, even if only in spirit. The same way I hope his father and uncle will feel when I am not physically here, that they will be guided by the lessons I taught them and be good and honorable men.

My hope is that whenever anyone thinks of me,

they will smile at a particular memory of time we shared together, or how I might have helped them in some way.

When it comes to thriving, I am reminded of one of my favorite TV shows, *"The West Wing."* In it, the character who plays President Jeb Bartlett, Martin Sheen often says "what's next?" to his staff after they complete an important meeting or policy negotiation. That should be how you live your life after you first survive cancer, and then thrive in your life after cancer, *what's next?*

What will you do differently? What are some of the things you had been putting off that now you feel is the right time to get started. A motivational speaker I know, Larry Winget, used to use the phrase "T-N-T", in his presentations, which stood for "Today Not Tomorrow." That's how I want you to start living your life, for today, not tomorrow. Because tomorrow is promised to no one.

If you notice I italicized the word "Thriver" in the title of this chapter.

You just looked back at the chapter title, didn't you? Dictionary.com defines italicizing as follows: *"Most commonly, italics are used for emphasis or contrast — that is, to draw attention to some particular part of a text."*

For the purpose of this chapter, I did it for emphasis. I wanted to emphasize that there is so much more to life, my life, your life, our lives than to just simply survive it.

Live it.

Get out there and do the things you have been putting off for too long waiting for the right time. Waiting to have enough money. Waiting for what I don't know. Waiting, waiting, waiting. Just do it.

Thrive!

Goals

I have always been a goal-oriented person. I set them, I achieve them, and then I make another. I was digging through some old boxes from college recently and found something that I knew I had to share in this chapter. In my senior year I took a Philosophy class and the professor assigned us a unique assignment. We had to create a quote that we would follow for the rest of our lives. The quote had to be original from us. We couldn't just take a variation of something someone else said and reword it. It had to be original.

We had about two weeks to complete the assignment and every night in my dorm room I just stared at a blank piece of paper, but nothing came. If it did, it sounded like something someone famous would say. I thought about my life and how I lived it and how every time I achieved a certain milestone or goal I would start again, not one to rest on my laurels. Finally, about two days before the assignment was due, I finally got it, and it read like this:

**"You must make a goal for yourself.
Once you accomplish this goal, you are not done.
You must make another, and ... GO FOR IT!"**

Jim Gano, 1983

Yep, I even signed it and dated it so that if I ever became famous and people started to quote this, they would know who said it and when.

This quote sums up how I have lived my whole life. In high school it might have been to catch a pass in a football game on Saturday. Or to finish a book report when it was due.

In my professional life there have been many goals that I have worked toward, maybe a promotion or salary level, or landing a new account, or running my own business and I would work toward those goals and once reached, I would make another and go for it.

So, my college quote really was just a summation of where I was in life at that time. But the funny thing is, as I look over my entire life, that is exactly how I have been living my whole life. Make a goal, accomplish a goal, make another. Rinse, lather, repeat.

You can feel free to use and quote my quote often, just tell people a really smart guy said it once back in 1983. (Oh, and tell them I was good looking too).

During my cancer journey there were a ton of goals I set for myself that were mostly short term. On a weekly basis there was the goal of getting through my chemo treatments and still returning to work that same day.

Then my calendar started to fill up with more and more appointments, and treatments, and I realized that most of my goals were now date driven and of short duration. I wasn't really planning for life after cancer.

At one point I had to tell my kids what was going on when I was finally diagnosed. My oldest son, Brandon had his own business right next door to mine so I called him up and asked him to come over. I remember this conversation like it was yesterday. Not for the tears and worry I thought he might display, but for what he said next.

After I told him about my diagnosis and treatment plan, he said to me "What are your goals?" He asked me again and I said, "I'd like to be back announcing football this fall." (I have been announcing our local high school football and basketball games for over 40 years.)

He said, "Too short. Make another one."

I replied "I want to be healthy enough to go to Angela's (my niece) wedding."

"Too short," came his reply once again.

In frustration I told him I have always worked toward goals and this had served me well, so why wasn't this good enough for him now? He said he had just read a book about goal setting and in it the author mentioned how sick people and people with cancer might make a goal like living long enough to see their daughter or son get married, or to witness the birth of a grandchild and once that happens, they die within six months. This was due to them putting all their energy into that one date, but not having anything to work toward after it had passed.

He told me I had to make long-term goals and think of them every day. I could still have the short-term goals of football and the wedding, but I had to have one goal that was years out. He said, "your goal should be to attend Brayden's wedding." At the time Brayden was my three-year-old grandson so what he was getting me to do was to think about something twenty to twenty-five years away. He wanted me to think about this day every day until it happened, because it would program my mind and body into focusing on long term things and not short term. This way if I achieved a short-term goal, my body and brain wouldn't think I could just stop. To this day I think about Brayden's wedding every day.

He's five now.

I have also started to make other long-term goals, things like vacations, eventual retirement, a trip to Nashville to see the Grand Ole Opry, and many more. The thing is I am no longer living just to get through a certain day, or week, or month, rather I am still doing those things and accomplishing the short-term goals while working toward my long-term ones.

What about you? Have you stopped thinking long term and given up on doing what you always wanted to do because of your diagnosis. Set a long-term goal, like a vacation. Research the costs, the travel, the places you will stay.

Get your finger off the damned pause button and plan on living your life once you beat cancer. Then send me a post card from wherever you go!

The shortest conversation

When I was going through my Stem cell transplant there were a lot of people who would enter my room. Obviously, there was the usual parade of doctors and nurses and technicians, but others would stop in as well, Nutritionists, Dietician's and Social Workers.

Each had a job to do and would go over their material with me in great detail. It was a meeting with a social worker that I remember best. She came in and in a very calm, soothing voice introduced herself and asked me how I was doing. I said, "great." It was as if she was expecting me to be forlorn, or depressed.

She handed me some papers and started right in with her presentation, "I'd like to talk to you about how you are handling the five stages of grief since your diagnosis."

I asked her, "Why?"

She said, "Well when you receive a cancer diagnosis there is a certain loss if you will, and you may need help processing that."

If you are not familiar, the five stages of grief are: denial, anger, bargaining, depression and acceptance.

I told her, "There is only one stage that matters to me right now and that is acceptance. I can't deny that I have cancer, I could be angry about it, but won't because that's just wasted energy, I can't bargain my way out of cancer with anyone, getting depressed about it will not help me and simply is not in my DNA, which leaves us with acceptance. I've accepted that I have cancer, now I have to focus all my energies on getting rid of it."

She looked at me for a long moment and said, "I blocked out forty-five minutes for this conversation, but I get the feeling I won't be here that long."

I said, "I'm not trying to be rude, but what I just said is how I feel. I've come to terms with it. The rest, to me, is just wasted energy. My job is to focus on getting better. Going through this process and moving on."

She said, "I don't think I've ever met anyone with your attitude toward their diagnosis." We talked for a few more minutes and then she left. She did stop by to check in on me a few more times during my two-week stay and each time my answer was the same. She had even talked to my nurses to see if I was putting on an act when she came in the room and they all said no, that I was that way with everyone.

Don't get me wrong, for some people it is perfectly normal to experience all five stages of grief when they receive their diagnosis. Sometimes though they get stuck on one or another for too long. If you deny you have cancer for too long and don't start treatment, you are only allowing the cancer to grow further until it may be too late.

What will getting angry at having cancer do for you? It will make you miserable all day long and this will have an adverse effect on your relationship with others.

You absolutely cannot bargain your way out of this diagnosis. You've got it, now you have to deal with it. Who would you be bargaining with anyway? And what would you have to offer in return?

Yes, you can get depressed. Receiving the news that you have cancer is probably one of the worst pieces of information you can ever get. But, wallowing in that depression, much like anger, will not serve you well in the long run.

Finally, you can do what I did and accept your diagnosis and then create a plan with your medical team on how it will be treated and hopefully cured, or put into remission (hopefully for a long time).

The five stages of grief and how one responds to them are equally applicable to both the patient and the caregiver. You both are going through this. Some, like me, will respond differently than others, so you have to support one another through each of the stages. Everybody will respond differently so be there for one another. Talk it out about how you are feeling, your hopes, your fears and in some cases the inevitable. What if the treatment(s) don't work?

Respect each other's feelings and fears and for

the caregiver it is okay for you to seek counsel from someone else. I don't think it is healthy for it to be just you and the person you are caring for. You might need to lean on a friend to discuss things you can't, or won't discuss with the patient.

My wife is one of the strongest women I know, but a couple nights before I was admitted she said something that rocked me to my core because in all our time together she had never said these words. She said, "I'm scared." Before I went into the hospital for my two-week stay for the transplant, I texted all of my wife's friends I had cell phone numbers for and asked them to check up on her while I was away. It was the first time I had ever heard her say she was scared about anything. I did the same with my kids. I was more worried about her, than I was me.

My wife has always been the worrier in the family, now here I was worried about her.

During my stay, again during the pandemic she was the only visitor I was allowed to have. She was also only allowed to visit for four hours a day and they had to be the same four hours, usually nine in the morning until one in the afternoon.

We live an hour away from the hospital so I know this was tough on her and I tried my best to be upbeat for her whenever she visited. Sometimes I was wiped out from the drugs, but did my best to stay awake for her so she wouldn't worry.

As my caregiver, and my wife, she was my ace in the hole. With her background in cancer research and bloodwork she could look at my labs and numbers and tell me how I was responding even before the doctors did.

If you don't have a spouse or significant other

or friends that can be there for you and help get you to appointments or make sure you have food in the house, find someone, anyone who will, maybe a co-worker you are friendly with, just don't go it alone.

And as soon as you can, find acceptance.

Motivations

This is one of my favorite topics. Motivations. What motivates you? What motivates me? There are times both before I had cancer, during treatment, and now after when I needed a little extra motivation to get through my day, or a particular task. So where do I find it? Everywhere. I can be motivated by a famous quote, by music, by movie scenes. You name it and I can be motivated by it. I even have some "go to" motivators that I will play whenever I need a little push.

A simple one and one almost everyone knows, is the song *"Eye of the Tiger"* by Survivor, the theme from the Rocky movies. That is one song that will get my blood pumping, also listening to *"Crazy Train"* by Ozzy Osbourne.

Sometimes, I can be motivated by famous

quotes or passages like the aforementioned *"Man in the Arena"* by Teddy Roosevelt.

Sit me down to watch the locker room speech by Kurt Russell as Coach Herb Brooks of the 1980 Miracle on Ice hockey team in the movie *"Miracle,"* and I'll be ready to take on the Russians myself.

Do you have any motivators? It can be anything like I said from literature, to famous quotes, to scripture, to music to favorite scenes from a favorite TV show or movie. Anything that gets you going and makes you want to take on the world.

My other favorite motivators are my business and my family and not necessarily in that order. I don't want to see my business fail because I have/had cancer or due to having to close because of the pandemic. When the pandemic hit, businesses were forced to close for "two weeks" in New Jersey and particularly in my industry with schools closed and everyone working from home and no sports activities, or corporate events going on, my business really suffered, for two years.

I felt as if I was fighting an invisible foe. Much the same way I feel about cancer. The punches kept coming, but I couldn't see my opponent. If another business moved into my town and sold the same products I do at a better price, with better quality and offered better customer service I would acknowledge that they had beaten me, but with COVID and cancer I could not see my opponent(s). But I had to keep fighting.

It was hard to get up every day after laying off my entire staff and going to work and literally doing everything I could to keep the business open. There were many pivots along the way, but somehow, I did it. And you can bet the soundtrack of music in my truck and my production area was pumping with a lot of upbeat music to help get me through the day.

There were even times when I would have to go into my office, get on YouTube and watch the Miracle speech, just to reset my mindset. Or maybe my favorite dogfight scenes from the Top Gun movies.

The same holds true with my family. I have always been there for my kids and wanted to do the same with my Grandkids. For the first two years of his life my son brought his son, my grandson, to work with him almost every day. I got to share in some of the care like bottle feeding, diaper changing, and as he got older reading books to him. He was with me every day to the point where I hated weekends because unless we were going to visit them, I would have to wait 48 hours to see him again.

He and I grew very close and have a very special bond. At four years old he figured out how to use his mother's phone to have video calls with me, and I have to tell you there is nothing better than seeing his face on my screen saying "Hi, Pop Pop!" Puts a big old smile on my face every time. Now we are doing the calls with his two sisters as well.

Talk about motivators. During my cancer journey I realized that if I was no longer around, how would they remember me. Would they remember me? Or, would I just be a picture in a photo album or picture frame and when they asked "who's that?" someone would just say "Oh, that's your grandfather, daddy's dad."

Nope. Cancer was not going to take that away from me. Not if I had anything to do with it. When I was at my lowest, we would settle for phone calls, because I didn't want the kids to see me looking bad. Once I started to recover, we resumed our video calls.

I feel as if I have much to teach them. I so want to watch them grow into young men and women and it fascinates me now how much they change from week to week. I cherish the drawings they would make me that said "We love you, Pop Pop!" when I was going into the hospital, and still have them to this day. They are in fact still motivators for me.

Now, they live a few states away but when we can get away, my wife and I drive down and visit them. We tell their parents do what you have to do and we'll watch after the kids. I teasingly call these 'working vacations.'

To show you how intuitive kids are, my grandson knew when my back was hurting while I was wearing the back brace. A few months after the Kyphoplasty procedures to fix my back and after I had finished my transplant we were playing in his backyard. I picked him up and gave him a piggy back ride back to the house, something that would have been impossible just a few months earlier.

When we approached the house, I put him down. He grabbed my hand and stopped me, then looked up to me and said "Pop Pop, that doctor sure did a good job fixing your back."

Motivators.

I keep a small journal type notebook that I have kept for years, and when I hear or read a quote that inspires me, or motivates me, I write it down in there. Then when I need a good kick in the pants, I'll read a few of them. Every now and then you can catch me searching the internet for motivational quotes. I also host a weekly radio show/podcast and start the show with the "Quote of the Week" which is usually a quote meant to inspire my audience.

Regardless of what you choose to motivate

yourself, whether it be music, quotes, movies, or family or something else, keep looking for new ones that you can add to your library. There are days when some of my tried-and-true motivators just aren't enough, so I look for new ones.

I am a sports minded person, and played sports most of my life, I love some of the famous quotes that coaches or athletes will say when they describe the competition or a tough game just won, or even how they handle defeat, so I write those down.

Sometimes, a lyric in a song will resonate with me so I write down the title so I can listen to it again, or try to memorize the lyric. As a peer mentor volunteer with the Cancer Hope Network I share some of these with the people I am mentoring, fellow cancer patients going through treatment and they all tell me they love them.

There are those who might say "you make it sound so easy," and let me assure you I am not trying to do that in any way. I am sharing with you what works/worked for me. I know it's hard, I know how taxing it is physically, mentally and emotionally. I am not in denial in any way. But I am a fighter, always have been, and I will not let an invisible foe like cancer beat me.

Regardless of what stage of grief you might be in, try to find something, anything that motivates you to keep pressing on. To push yourself through the hard times so that hopefully you will achieve success down the road.

The most surprising question

A couple of years ago I met a couple who had lost their daughter at the age of 13. She had endured six open heart surgeries and finally succumbed to a rare form of cancer. They asked me for some help creating some awards for a fundraiser they were having to benefit the foundation they had established in their daughter's name, Marisa.

When they came to pick up the awards they asked for the bill and I said there wasn't one. They couldn't believe it and were genuinely very thankful. They left the store and I thought that would be it. The husband who used to be a reporter for a local newspaper called me up a few days later and said he wanted to have a story written about me and all I do in the community helping various organizations and especially those geared toward the Autism community. I agreed to do the interview and he sent over a reporter to talk to me.

We talked for an hour and a half as he asked me question after question about me, my business, my community involvement, etc. But it was his last question that really threw me for a loop. More on this in a minute but I want to give you a little background as it pertains to this story.

Back in college I had taken a course called "Death and Dying." Funny how I'm writing a book about how I survived cancer and am talking about a school subject like that. It was taught by a local priest who was on faculty at the school. One of his assignments was for us to write our own obituary. Actually, we had to write two. One would be if we died today (keep in mind we were around twenty at the time) and one would be if we had lived into our eighties.

This was one of the toughest assignments I'd ever received. Why? Because I didn't think I had done anything yet. Up until this point in my life all I felt I had done was grow up, go to school, play sports, etc. The typical things most kids did. The most I had ever done was served as a volunteer at the local hospital and with the Special Olympics.

At best, my obituary of where I was in my life to that point might fill two paragraphs. The second part of the assignment was for us to imagine we were in our eighties and what we thought we might accomplish in the next sixty years. How would we be remembered. Of course, there were no right or wrong responses you were just making things up as you went along.

We wrote the typical things about being married, having kids, our made-up career which for some tracked with what they were studying, maybe some volunteer activities or accomplishments, and then when and where our services would be held.

When we were done, he said something that has always stuck with me. He said, "Live every day as if you are writing your obituary." When asked what he meant by that he replied "How do you want to be remembered? What will you accomplish in your life that will make people take pause and remember or think of you long after you are gone. Generationally, your children will remember you, their children may have a few memories of you, but in one-hundred years, your own descendants will have very little knowledge of who you are, or what you did during your lifetime."

Way to bring us all down father. But it did get me to thinking, and it motivated me in some way that I don't think I ever thought about or realized until the reporter asked me his question.

His last question to me which really made me think was, "If I were to look up your Wikipedia™ page, what would it say about you?" Hmmm, that will get you thinking. It was sort of like the priest's obituary exercise. Keep in mind I've written for newspapers and magazines, worked in radio and television so I was used to being the one asking the tough questions, not answering them, and this one really caught me off guard.

I replied, "I don't have a Wikipedia page."

He said, "I know. I checked, but if you did, what would it say about you?"

I said, "I hope it would say I was a good husband, father and friend, also a good businessman. That I helped people where and when I could and that

I was a hard worker."

He answered, "There has to be more that, just with what I've learned about you in the last ninety or so minutes I know there is more than that."

I stared at him for a long time, maybe thirty or more seconds. During this time, I thought about my life as I had never thought about it before, then I said, "I hope that my Wikipedia page would say something like "He made a difference in many people's lives."

He replied, "That's it. I just wanted to hear you say it, because it appears based on my research of you, you live that way every day."

The fact is I truly do live my life like that every day. I know I have been blessed with a great family and friends. I want others to have that too. My employees and people I come in contact with who are struggling. Sometimes it is a simple word of encouragement or sitting them down to map out what they can do to be successful. I have a drawer full of cards and letters from people who tell me I've inspired them to make a necessary change that has brought them career, or financial success. I love when people write to me letters like that because it shows I am doing what I think I was always meant to do, help people.

Hopefully, one hundred years from now someone will still reference my name and they will recognize the difference I made in someone's life they knew.

Clear Eyes. Full Heart. Can't Lose.

If you've ever seen the movie or TV show Friday Night Lights, you probably recognize that phrase. *"Clear Eyes, Full Heart, Can't Lose."* This simple sentence becomes the mantra of the Dillon Panthers football team and it became mine as well.

I even had tee shirts made up with that phrase on the front of the shirt and the words "I'm Not Done Yet!" on the back. I had three of these shirts made up and brought them with me to the hospital. I still wear them to my follow-up appointments.

The nurses loved these shirts and some have even asked me to make one for them. When I asked them why they say, "So many people come here with a defeatist attitude, but not you. You have been clear eyes and full heart from day one. You are a refreshing change from the normal patient we see and interact with on a daily basis."

Maybe I am wired differently than everybody else, I don't know. But I have always been very upbeat, with a positive mental attitude and an optimist. I remember one time I was coaching my son's hockey team and we were down by three goals with about three minutes to play. I called a timeout and said, "Guys, I once saw the Philadelphia Flyers score three goals in 35 seconds, you can do this if you work like a team and believe in each other." Heck, we had three minutes. On the first faceoff we scored in eleven seconds. The next faceoff we scored in twenty. My players were looking at me like I was a genius. It took a little longer but we scored the third goal to tie the game just before time ran out. Then we won in overtime.

Clear Eyes. Full Heart. Can't Lose.

How does that saying relate to a guy or girl with cancer. I had just finished rewatching Friday Night Lights on Netflix before my diagnosis so it was still rattling around in my brain when I found out.

Clear Eyes. – To me this meant I had to focus. Focus on me, my disease, my treatment. I now had to become a student again. It also meant I had to let a few things go in my life like sitting on certain Boards of Directors and my favorite thing in life, announcing Panther Basketball games at Bridgewater-Raritan High School. That really hurt because I enjoyed it so much and had been doing it for so long. When I put down the microphone, I told our Athletic Director "Keep my seat warm, I'll be back." To which he said that chair was mine for as long as I wanted it. It made my cancer real to me. I had to focus on me. As my wife said, I had to learn to say the word "No" to people. The hospital I go to for labs has a portal and will email you when certain tests are in your chart. I had to learn what these numbers meant. I remember telling the doctor that even though I get the results I don't always know what they mean (my wife did, I didn't). His Nurse Practitioner looked right at me and said "Don't worry in six months you'll be an expert in all of them." For the most part she was right. I'll admit at first, I cheated and would Google "what does a low WBC POC blood level mean?" then I would confer with my wife to verify if this was something serious.

The way my doctor sets up his appointments is you go to the hospital one week for labs then schedule a visit with him for the following week. By the time I meet with him I already know how I'm doing and if anything is too abnormal. My wife and I will go into these appointments with very specific questions about certain blood markers. Once these questions were answered by the doctor, we were able to rest easy for a while. A week later we would repeat the same labs with the transplant team at another hospital and once I received the all clear I didn't have to think about cancer for another three months.

It always amazes me how I can put cancer on the back burner so easily for a period of time, then when I see I have a doctor appointment coming up on my calendar I get anxious. Remember that little gray cloud?

Full Heart. – To me this meant surrounding myself with those I love. My family and friends, at least those who stuck around. I am on the Hall of Fame Committee at my high school and working on our annual induction ceremony dinner kept me busy during my hospital stay and I only hoped I would be ready and healthy enough to emcee the dinner that October. That goal, or as I called it "10/22/22" (the date of the induction dinner) kept me pushing hard to regain my strength and stamina. When I met with the doctors, I would tell them "10/22/22" and when they asked what that meant I would say, "That is the date you have to get me better by." All of the things I enjoy, my family, my work, my volunteer activities you could lump into the full heart bucket.

When a friend, colleague or family member would write, text or call me my heart was full. If my grandkids told me they loved me on the phone, my heart was full. Seeing my wife make the daily trip to the hospital just so she could sit in the room with me, made my heart full.

This fullness in my heart has not left, and it really pisses me off to think how much of my life I took for granted before my diagnosis. I never once thought about what it would be like for some of these people if I wasn't here. I never thought of all I would miss if I wasn't here. Man, if you need something to motivate you into getting better, stew on those thoughts for a few minutes.

Can't Lose. – Finally, there is "Can't Lose." This was perhaps the most important part of this saying. I couldn't lose this fight. I couldn't give in to cancer and check out at the age of sixty or sixty-one. There was still too much living for me to do. I want to take my wife back to Italy, drink wine and eat pasta again.

My first step toward 'can't lose' was when I surprised my wife with a river cruise to Europe that I planned for the one-year anniversary of being told I was in remission. We travelled with some friends and as we stepped off the plane I walked in front of my wife by a few steps because I didn't want her to see the tears that were streaming down my face. Happy tears.

I made it.

I still wasn't in the best physical shape for the amount of walking we would be doing, but I "powered through it" and enjoyed every minute of that trip.

I 'refused to lose' as Ray Evernham might say to cancer and I met my first long range goal post treatment. There is still so much more I want, and need to do, and I am already working on that. I do have to listen to my body as sometimes I get a little too tired, or too sore and need to rest, but once I feel better it's time to get back in this game we call life. It's time to start planning another trip soon. It's time for some more Pici pasta in Italy!

And I'll do it with Clear Eyes, a Full Heart, and a Can't Lose mentality.

You're Done

As I mentioned earlier after the Stem cell transplant, I had to receive every childhood vaccination in one-third doses every three months for the next two years. Finally, the day of my last appointment arrived. We reviewed my bloodwork numbers and the Nurse Practitioner asked if we had any questions.

To say I had been waiting for this day for a long time would be an understatement. For the previous two years I had been poked and prodded and tested and I was tired of seeing doctors. To be honest although I will never be able to thank them enough, I was getting tired of driving an hour north to see them.

The reason for this is if you've ever driven on Route 80 in Northern, New Jersey you know it's like driving down Main Street in Baghdad. If the cancer doesn't kill you, the way that road shakes your teeth and vital organs just might.

When the Nurse Practitioner closed her laptop, she looked up at me and said, "Okay, you're done."

I asked, "What does that mean, you're done."

She said, "You've received all your vaccinations, you are still in remission, from now on you can just follow up with your Hematology/Oncology doctor at Morristown and if something changes, they can always loop us back in."

I said, "No."

She asked, "What did you say?"

I said, "No. I like you guys and it gives me a sense of comfort and calm when you tell me I'm doing okay. I can look at the blood numbers and see I'm all good, but when I hear it from you, it puts me at ease."

Funny how just a few paragraphs ago I was telling you how I couldn't wait to be done with these people, huh?

I asked her if in fact I could keep coming and she said yes and made an appointment for me now six months out. I also verified that insurance would pay for it and she said yes.

I don't know why, but I was actually scared when she said I was done. Maybe that one person was right and we do have some level of PTSD, but hearing her say I was done really affected me. I don't know why it is so important for me to hear from them that I am okay. I assume it has something to do with the fact that there is a good chance I wouldn't be here if it weren't for them. Either way, I'm glad I get to go back, and now I know I should try to move away from them, which is what I originally wanted to do, until they said I could.

Money, Money, Money ...

What a great song by the 1970's group ABBA. In the song there is a line that goes,

"Money, money, money
Must be funny
In the rich man's world
Money, money, money
Always sunny
In the rich man's world
All the things I could do
If I had a little money
It's a rich man's world..."

Why am I talking about money? Because in this country the insurance mechanism is broken and as a cancer patient with the high costs of drugs and various treatments you could find yourself bankrupt in a matter of months if you don't know how to navigate the system.

Here is my story and I have shared this with many cancer patients that simply don't know there are other ways to pay for medicine. When my chemo treatments started, I was placed on a drug (Revlimid) that could only be obtained through what was called a "specialty pharma" company.

It had to be delivered carefully, handled carefully, women of child bearing years couldn't touch it, and the first dose, which would last for one month cost me ninety dollars ($90.00). Sounds simple, right?

The following month it was time for the renewal of the prescription and during this time my father-in-law had died. The company called me to authorize the reorder of the prescription and said they would gladly accept payment before shipping. I thought it would be ninety dollars again and reached for my wallet in my pocket to retrieve my credit card. Then the woman on the phone said that it would be Eleven Thousand Six-Hundred dollars ($11,600.00)! She then asked if I wanted to put that on my credit card as if I was buying a shirt from L.L. Bean. Keep in mind, I have great medical insurance and this drug was not covered.

Yep, you read that right. When I asked why so much, they said the first payment was an introductory rate, but this is what I would be paying as long as I was on the drug. Since I was scheduled to be on it at least 4-5 months my head was spinning thinking of spending over fifty thousand dollars for this medication.

I told the woman I would have to call her back and was prepared, in my head anyway, to cease all treatments right then and there. There was no way I was going to bankrupt my family.

Without thinking I called my wife. I forgot that she was out with her brothers searching for a place to hold a repast luncheon after their father's funeral. I told her, (she was on speakerphone), how much the medicine was going to cost and you could hear everyone in that car audibly gasp and then say "WHAT?!"

My wife said she would make some phone calls and call me back, but that I should not pay that sum. My wife called the patient help line at the manufacturer and after describing my situation was able to negotiate the price down to fifty dollars ($50.00) per refill.

The question I have is why do these companies put the patient through that kind of angst? If you know you can charge fifty dollars, charge the fifty dollars. But Eleven Thousand Six hundred? That is unacceptable.

Having been married to a woman who has worked in cancer research I fully understand the costs associated with developing a drug to bring it to market. I get it. But, if you can offer to reduce my contribution down to fifty dollars, why don't we start there?

I mentioned earlier that I am on a forum page on Facebook for patients with Multiple Myeloma and I cannot tell you how many people have described going through a similar experience either for the same drug or a different one.

One man told the story of how he would have to remortgage or sell his home, had maxed out his credit cards and was looking to take a loan out to pay for his drugs.

It absolutely baffles me why we put cancer

patients or anyone with a chronic illness through this. As if they don't have enough to process with getting a diagnosis of a horrible disease, beginning treatment and then facing charges that could bankrupt them. The stress level goes through the roof.

The next time you are watching television and one of those drug commercials comes on listen carefully and read the fine print on the bottom of the screen. The announcer will usually say something like "If you can't afford your medication, (insert company name here) may be able to help." There will usually be a website or toll-free number you can contact for financial assistance. That is a call worth making if it means you can save thousands of dollars on the cost of your prescription.

I often wonder how many people did not know there were programs to help the patient offset the costs of these drugs? How many people have lost their homes or taken on considerable debt to pay for medications that could have been offset by the companies?

There are grants through other organizations as well, but they come up on an irregular basis so you pretty much have to monitor their websites daily to see if the window is open.

Ask your case manager if they know of any programs or grants that can help offset the cost of medications or treatments. Additionally, find out who the manufacturer of the drug is and call their patient care line. Most companies have these and are willing to help, unfortunately, you have to be the one to ask.

Then once you have some hard data on costs, contact your congressman or woman and explain to them the hardship and impact these exorbitant costs have had on you and your family.

Finally, if you do get some help from an organization or a manufacturer, thank them. The attitude of gratitude here can go a long way in encouraging these folks to keep these programs running for the next patient.

Your Bucket List

A long time ago, I used to be a person that would scribble on a notepad different things I wanted to do. Go to a Bruce Springsteen concert, check. Write and publish a book, check and check, this one will count as my third check. Have my name appear in liner notes on a music album, Check, and thanks Colt Ford. Meet and interview various celebrities, too many checks to include here. It was a bucket list if you will, but I don't do that anymore. I still have many things I want to do, but I stopped putting them on a "bucket list."

I have a friend who has a very detailed "dream list" the things she dreams of doing before she dies. Her list is even numbered in order of importance.

In 2007 there was a movie starring Jack

Nicholson and Morgan Freeman called "The Bucket List" and I suspect this is when everyone started making their lists. In the movie, Morgan Freeman explains to Jack Nicholson that the piece of paper he found lying on the floor is his "Bucket list." A list of things he wanted to do before he, you know, kicked the bucket.

I guess mine was a bucket list too, but I don't write anything on it anymore. Now I have what I call a "Do It Now" list.

C'mon Jim there has to be something you want to do? You might be asking, and you'd be right. There are a lot of things I want to do. I just don't put them on a list anymore. Now, if I want to do something, I do it. I'll figure out what it is I want to do, how much it will cost, when I can fit it into my schedule, and then I will do it.

This attitude was all mine before I was diagnosed, but perhaps heightened by the diagnosis. I am probably the hardest person to shop for at Christmas, because if I see something I like in June, I probably buy it then, typically a new tool for my shop. Why would I wait six months to ask for it from Santa Claus when I might need it then to complete a project.

I am a huge NASCAR fan and years ago I had the opportunity to drive a real NASCAR race car at the Richard Petty Driving Experience on a since demolished, one-mile Tri-Oval racetrack in Orlando, Florida. We flew down there for a vacation and we had a one-day detour to the racetrack. I had even borrowed a friend's pick-up truck for a week before we left, so I could reteach myself how to shift as I hadn't driven a manual transmission car in years.

I sat in on the prep class, got fitted for my driving suit and helmet, then we made our way to the track. I slid into the car and got buckled in. This may sound weird, but in the moments before we started the engines the only thing I could hear was my breathing, and my heartbeat in my ears in the helmet.

The next thing I knew we got the command to fire the engines and rolled off pit road. We took two caution laps to get the engines up to temperature and then they dropped the green flag. I put the hammer down and I was driving the fastest I had ever driven in my life. If someone had a microphone on me, they probably would have heard me laughing. I was loving every minute of it.

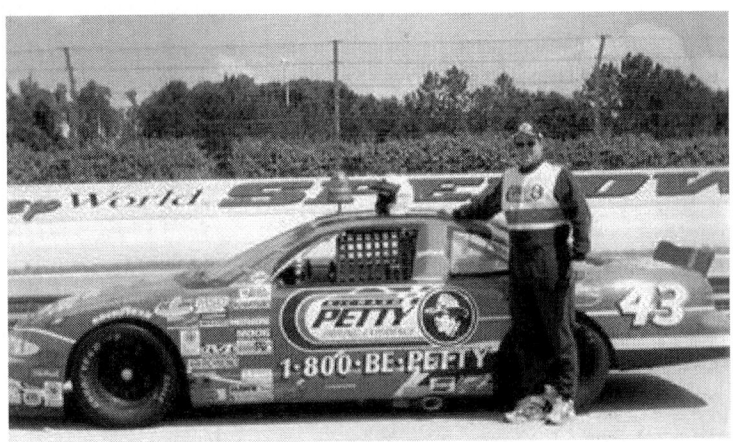

Me pictured at the Richard Petty Driving experience getting ready to turn some hot laps.

After ten hot laps we came into the pits for a quick debrief. They showed me my lap times and I was around 135 miles per hour. They told me how I could go faster and to trust the car. The cool thing was it felt like the car was velcroed to the racing surface. I don't think I've ever had that much traction in a passenger vehicle or truck that I've driven. My instructor encouraged me to hit my marks and try to go faster.

Out we went again and this time I got it up to a

155 mile per hour average. As bucket list items go, this was and has been at the very top for me. I have been fortunate to do other things and experiences I wanted to do and there are more yet to be done. However, I'm not going to stare at a piece of paper when I'm on the porch at the old folk's home, I'll be telling people all the cool things I did when I could.

The point here is simple, we only have so many days on this earth, so enjoy them. Do the things you want to do. Don't long for them and dream about them, do them. And do them now while you can. If you are currently in treatment maybe some things on your list will have to wait until you are better. Once you are, you'd better get to it, because times a wastin'.

I saw a cute cartoon the other day that kind of put this in perspective. Two old grandmotherly type women were sitting on a bench. One of them was holding a piece of paper while the other one said, "What's that?"

The one with the paper replied, "It's my bucket list."

The first woman replied "change the B to an F and you'll feel much better."

Whether you decide to maintain a bucket list or switch to my version, the "Do It Now" list, or the "F*$& it" list like the old lady suggested, never stop living your life, don't put it on pause for anyone or anything and never stop dreaming of all you can do.

But do start doing it.

Filling the Dash

Around my house, or at work, if people ask me what I am doing I might often respond with "I'm filling the dash." Some people know what I am referring to, others do not, so I'll explain it to you.

When we die, there will be a headstone with our name on it. Below that will be two dates, the date we are born and the date we died. But in between the dates will be a dash. To me that dash represents your life story. Everything you do every day is represented by that dash.

It could represent your work, your volunteer activities, being a parent or friend, holiday gatherings, vacations you have taken and memories you have made. Everything you do, every experience you have done will be represented by the dash.

When I am announcing a football or basketball game at my local high school, I am filling the dash. When I am running my business, I'm filling the dash. Even writing this book I am filling the dash. When I work with special needs kids to teach them job and life skills in my business, I am filling the dash. Even when I was going through treatment for cancer I was, you guessed it, filling the dash.

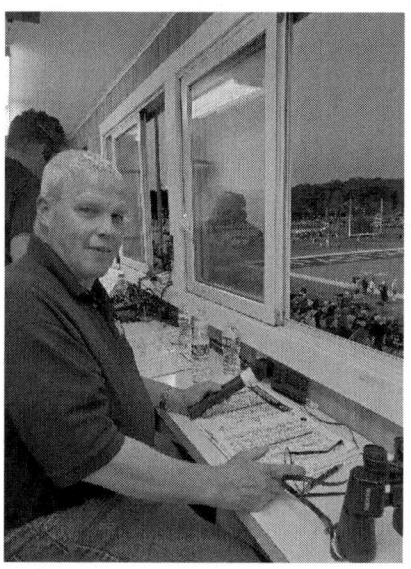

I did it! Back in the press box after my Stem cell transplant for my first game of the year.

And you can too. Life does not stop when you or a loved one receives a cancer diagnosis. You hopefully can still attend family functions like weddings and birthdays when your condition permits.

You can take small day trips, go out to lunch when your appetite allows you to.

The point is simple. Keep living your life. I've known some people who have led some tremendous lives, but once they are diagnosed with cancer it's as if all they are doing is waiting to die. They had lost that fire within that had motivated them for so long. They were in the denial stage of the five stages of grief and could not pull themselves out of it.

And don't listen to the statistics. When you read "the average survival rate is XX years" you have to question a few things. When was this written? What therapies were available then? Is it from a reputable source and backed up by clinical data?

My doctors have told me that as little as ten years ago a diagnosis of Multiple Myeloma was like a death sentence with a three-to-five-year survival rate. What they also tell me is there has been so much research and new therapies coming out including Stem Cell and CAR-T therapies that now they no longer treat it as a cancer, rather they think of it as a chronic disease. Ideally you are diagnosed with it, get treated, obtain remission, either go on maintenance drugs, or not, and continue on with your life. They have told me that eventually in most patients it will return and we have many tools in our toolbox with which to fight it again and hopefully achieve remission again.

I am encouraged by the amount of research being done and the new announcements being made about great progress being achieved in human clinical trials that could result in even more treatments and hopefully one day, a cure for most cancers.

While the doctors and clinicians continue their research, I am continuing to live my life. Admittedly, there are some limitations physically, specifically with my back. But I try to adapt as best I can to continue doing the things I love. If I am ever unable to do something I love, like golf, then I'll find something else.

Where you won't find me is sitting at home, waiting to die. That is simply not in my DNA.

At the end of this book, I have included a beautiful poem that sums up what "filling the dash" is all about.

If you were to look back on your life pre-diagnosis, how would you say you filled your dash? Are you still doing that, or have you stopped? If so, why? Could you see yourself doing those activities again if they brought you joy? If so, then do them.

There are no pause buttons in the game of life.

Charlie Brown and Snoopy

When I was in the hospital, I was scrolling the internet one day for newspapers to read and I came upon a section of comics in one of the papers I read. It was a Peanuts™ cartoon and just one panel.

In it you see Charlie Brown and Snoopy sitting on a brick wall. You are looking at them from behind. Charlie Brown says to Snoopy, "You only live once Snoopy." To which his faithful companion replies, "No Charlie Brown, you only die once, you live every day."

BINGO! If ever there was a cartoon that would sum up my attitude for living and life, this was it. I love that cartoon. Two simple sentences that sum up exactly how I approach life. How many times have you heard someone say "you only live once," or use the

127

abbreviation "YOLO." I've even seen those letters on tee shirts. If that is the way you approach life you've got it all wrong and a beagle just proved it to you. Yes, we only have one life to live, but we get to live it every day.

In a previous chapter I talked to you about setting goals. Here is a little-known fact about me. Every night when I go to bed, I make a goal for myself and it is very simply to wake up the next morning. When six o'clock rolls around and the alarm goes off, I am already filled with a sense of accomplishment because I have already done the first thing I wanted to do that day!

You may say that is the stupidest thing I've ever read, but guess what when you do it a few times and realize how it makes you feel in the morning you'll start doing it too. Of course, one day I may not complete that goal, but I'm guessing it won't matter too much then.

Right now, where is your mindset? Are you thinking like Charlie Brown, or like Snoopy? Pre-diagnosis, did you have the same mindset. After reading Snoopy's quote did it change your thinking for a minute or two?

Are you living every day as Snoopy would want you to do? If not, why not? As I've said throughout this book, we don't know how many days we have on this earth. I hope for you there are many more sunrises and sunsets, but ask yourself are you truly living? Squeezing as much joy out of every day as you can. Even if you are going through treatment where many people tell me they have to put their life on hold, are you living? Are you doing anything just for you? It could be anything as long as it is about you.

Unfortunately, there is no pause button in life. It's not like a song on a tape where you can just hit pause and come back and listen to it later. No, life and time both march on, with or without you. So, take your finger off the pause button and get back to living. It may be a little harder depending on your condition but try to push yourself. I have many times here is one example.

I own a 1948 Plymouth Special Deluxe classic car similar to the one pictured on the front cover of this book. When I was laid up in treatment the gas tank sprung a leak and gasoline poured all over the garage floor. Ooh baby my wife was not happy about that. Because of the condition of my back and how I was feeling coming off treatment I didn't think I would be able to fix it. Every day I would leave the house and look at my car, nicknamed "Dolly" and think, "I've got to fix her."

About one year after my transplant, I was feeling pretty good physically and got down on the floor to see what would be involved in replacing the tank. I watched a few YouTube™ videos that showed me the process and I was ready to go. I found a new gas tank on eBay™ and all the accompanying parts and ordered them. Then one weekend I jacked the car up and began to remove the old gas tank. It was hard. This whole job should have taken me four hours to remove the tank and install a new one. Instead, it took me three hours to unloosen the old tank and then my body ran out of gas and I had to stop. I still hadn't removed the old tank. I listened to my body and I rested.

The next weekend I finally got the old one off, and started to install the new one. As with most after-market car parts it fought me every step of the way and after a few hours I was worn out and had to stop again.

Finally, on the third weekend I got it fitted in place and plumbed. I was so happy that I didn't give up and realized that yes, some tasks would take longer for me to do, but when you see me driving "Dolly" on Sunday afternoons, or at car shows that smile on my face tells you all you need to know about me, that I am truly in my happy place.

I also love to read and write, and certain chemo drugs really messed up my vision for around 6–8 months. I tried to compensate with drug store cheater glasses, but could only read for short periods of time. Still, I kept trying. Don't let your disease rob you of the things you enjoy.

There will be days when you can't do certain things, but there will also be days when you'll feel you can do anything. Don't waste those days.

When you go out to dinner order a drink, not too many, but enjoy yourself. Order dessert, you know you want it, enjoy it. No matter what you do, enjoy this life while you are in it.

My brother-in-law David used to recite a quote that goes along with the theme of this chapter when he said, *"Enjoy here while you're here, because there's no here, there."*

Wow. When you put it in that context, you can look at the balance in your 401k every day, but if you don't enjoy it while you're here what good is it? So, buy that dress you want. Hell, by the boat you want. Take the trip you've been dreaming of and wishing for. Do the things that will bring you joy. Don't deny yourself. Because like me you don't want to end up on the front porch of the old folks home saying "I coulda, I shoulda, I woulda."

Be like Nike and Just Do It.

Enjoy here, while you're here . . .

Survivor's Guilt

So far as you have read this story you might think I have had it easy during this cancer journey. It was not. I have left certain parts out of this book so as not to mire you in the details of some of the unpleasantries that go with cancer treatment. Trust me, I had to deal with all of them including nausea, a lot of nausea, getting sick, fatigue, night sweats, insomnia, uncontrollable muscle tremors, headaches, pain, diarrhea, constipation, you name it and I dealt with it. I just didn't think you wanted to read about all of that, but it was there during my treatments and thankfully I don't have to deal with it now.

I want to say, just as Lou Gehrig once said, "I consider myself the luckiest man on the face of the earth." But why? It's simple really. We started my treatment right away. I responded well. My Stem cell transplant was successful. I was declared in 'complete stringent remission.' I am on no maintenance drugs.

Yet so many people on the forum board I belong to on Facebook for Multiple Myeloma patients don't always have the same story. Some will complain about terrible neuropathy in their hands or feet. Others will tell stories about the side effects of certain maintenance drugs. Others have had months long bouts of either diarrhea or constipation from the drugs. Others depending on the drug they are taking will suffer through sleepless nights just as I did in the early stages of my chemo treatments.

I feel so bad for these individuals that their treatments could not have been as successful as mine. Who knows the cause. Were they diagnosed later than I was? Did they have co-morbidities that have compromised their body's ability to fight the disease? Is it their age? I don't know.

We are all encouraged to share our stories on the forum both good and bad. I think I suffer from 'survivor's guilt' when I read that someone is struggling, and I am not.

Occasionally, I will post something positive like the anniversary of my remission date. Or, the anniversary of my 're-birthday'. Many times, the comments section will be filled with thank you's from people telling me that my news has encouraged and inspired them to keep fighting, or that I give them hope and for that I am grateful.

But then I think about the people who did not leave a comment who may be sitting at home upset with my good fortune.

The worst news I can read on the board is that

one of our members on the forum page has lost their battle to this insidious disease, cancer and specifically, Multiple Myeloma. How can I post something positive when someone has just shared that a loved one has passed? I don't. I wait, until the subject matter becomes a little more positive, then I will share any good news I may have.

There was one post in particular that really resonated with me, because it was written by the woman who had the cancer and was posted for her by a friend shortly after she died. In it she spoke of her love for her family and friends and pets. She cursed the disease and thanked it all at the same time for opening her eyes to her own mortality. She thanked the members of the forum page for their encouragement and stories and encouraged all of us to keep fighting. It gave her time to write letters to her loved ones to be given to them upon her death and she admitted there were several of those.

I remember that my favorite line in her post was the last line. After she had written, quite beautifully I might add, her feelings about life and death she ended with one sentence when she said, *"and remember, eat dessert first."*

I sort of adopted that mentality. Why should I, or any of us for that matter deny ourselves the simple pleasures in life. So often when the waitress comes to the table after a meal they will ask, *"do you want any dessert or coffee?"* Invariably it seems everyone at the table will say, "no thank you." Deny, deny, deny. When deep down we're really saying, *"Ooh, that cheesecake sounds delicious,"* or *"I'm in the mood for ice cream."* Go for it. Order it and enjoy it, then think of her when you do.

What would my brother-in-law say? *"Enjoy here*

while you're here ..."

As I live my life and enjoy certain successes or milestones, I often think of all the people on that forum board who are no longer with us. And I think of the ones who are struggling with the management of their disease.

There is an old poem I remember that begins, *"Share with me my sadness and I'll share with you, my joy."* I think of that often as I read their posts and wish they could all share more joy. Just as I do. I love reading that a woman who was otherwise bedridden found the strength to tend to her garden one day. Or that a man who had been suffering was able to go to his workshop and create a gift for a grandchild out of wood. Then I can share any successes I might be having recently.

I do also share my setbacks, but there haven't been that many, but to keep it real I share them. Life isn't always rainbows and unicorns.

So many times though, I read the posts of the person who is struggling and I'll ask, "how did I get so lucky?" Yes, I had a great team of doctors and nurses. Yes, I had a great attitude and fighting spirit. So why did I do so well, and they did not? The answer never comes, and it bothers me.

I imagine this will continue for some time, but I also know that I am rooting for anyone dealing with cancer, any cancer, to have a successful outcome. I see the other patients in the waiting rooms and I can almost tell by the look in their eyes if they are newly diagnosed, or have been battling the disease for years, and I pray for them.

When I have mentioned this feeling to others who have had cancer they have told me they too have had these feelings, but they also say we paid the price by having to go through our treatments and we should celebrate our good fortune. Trust me, I am grateful. More than anyone can, or will, ever know. Still, it hurts me to see others suffer.

I'm not sure if any of you have felt this way and how you handled it. But hopefully you have found some solace in where you are right now.

Moving Day

I want to share with you a story about the goodness of people and how sometimes your good works can come back to benefit you.

I own my own business, and for the past 14 years I have worked with the local high school in bringing in special needs students to teach them job skills and life skills for twelve-week rotations through their Workplace Readiness Program. I love working with this program and seeing the progress the kids make in just a few weeks.

When I had the first compression fractures, I was in the process of getting ready to move my business. Our previous location had been deemed untenable due to black mold, a leaky roof and sewer back-ups. My older son who used to work with me offered to pay for the move as a Christmas present. We received one estimate for over thirty-eight hundred dollars ($3,800.00). I told him I appreciated the gesture, but there was no way I was going to let him pay that much money to move the business one mile down the road.

He said, "Let me work on it," and that was the last I heard of it for a while. A few months later he came into my office and said, "Be ready to move April first."

I said, "What do you mean?"

He replied, "I found a team of movers, and they're going to help us move."

I protested and said, "This better not be a bunch of day laborers, this equipment is expensive and they are not insured."

He said, "Don't worry about it, just be at the warehouse at eight o'clock on the first."

We pre-packed as much of our inventory as we could and then I waited for the first. I got up that morning, showered, put on that bulky back brace and drove to the office. When I drove behind the building to our parking area, my eyes started to tear up. Standing there next to a big yellow school bus were the students from the Workplace Readiness Program and their teachers and job coaches.

The lead teacher had heard about my cancer diagnosis and had called my son and asked "What can we do for your father? He has been so good to our program we want to do something."

So, they conspired and arranged to have the kids take a "field trip" to my store. Half the kids would stay there and load a box truck with all our things, the other half would go to the new location and arrange shelving systems and wait for the boxes to arrive, then put them in the correct place.

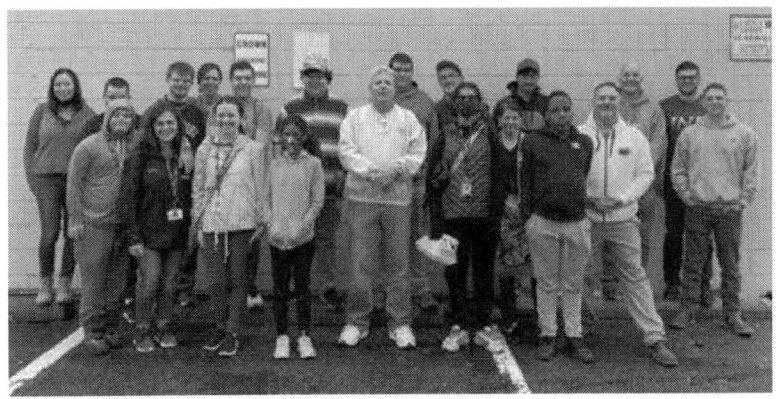

Students and teachers from the Workplace Readiness Program on "Moving Day"

It was a great day. The kids got to do some public service and give something back to someone who had helped build up their program and advocated for them in the community. All I had to do was sit in a chair and point to where I wanted the boxes to go. Instead of having to pay nearly four-thousand dollars to move, we only had to buy the kids sandwiches from Jersey Mike's™. Even some kids who graduated from the program came back to help!

Even now, a few years later when I see some of the kid's they'll remind me how much fun they had helping me move my business.

It was a lesson not only in the kindness of friends, but even the kindness of strangers, as I did not know all of the students who helped us move the business that day.

My Thank You

Military personnel, Police, Fire and EMS personnel often carry, or present, challenge coins to individuals in recognition or thanks of something.

A challenge coin is a uniquely designed coin that represents an organization or special occasion. Being given a challenge coin represents camaraderie, or unity, and proves membership of a certain group, as well as honoring the actions of those who receive them. We make these for several organizations at my business.

I was looking for a way to thank my many doctors, nurses, technicians, family members and friends for all of their support during my cancer journey. I had talked to many people and they said that often times patients might bring baked goods or something handmade as a display of their appreciation.

I am often asked to consult with small businesses to return them to profitability. This is usually done by an overhaul of their systems and marketing plans. When it comes to marketing, I often tell my clients *"You have to be different to be remembered."*

As I thought about that and how I would thank people who were there for me during my treatment those words kept ringing in my head. How could I be different? You probably wouldn't want me to bake you anything, or you might end up in the hospital again. I had no idea what I could make that would be memorable. And then it hit me.

I could design and have made a challenge coin. Something small that people could either carry in a purse, display on a desk, or for one friend with a military background display with the rest of his challenge coin collection.

As I sat in my hospital room, I took out a few sheets of paper and began to design my coin. On the front I knew I had to include my mantra phrase *"Clear Eyes. Full Heart, Can't Lose."* I then added my personal brand logo, my initials "JG" with two swooshes over them and finally a rope that wrapped all the way around the coin. I attached an index card with a typed message that explained each element of the coin.

I explained where the phrase Clear Eyes, Full Heart, Can't Lose came from, I explained about my personal brand, the initials that I use in my writing, and on my website, etc., an identifier if you will. Then I explained to them that the rope represented the ties that bind us together, whether as family, friend, or professional who took care of me and set me on the road to recovery.

On the obverse side of the coin, I added a burgundy awareness ribbon as that is the color of Multiple Myeloma awareness.

On the outer rim I included the words *"Thank you for all of your support"* on the top rocker, and my name on the bottom rocker. Then I wanted to show these people that their care, their prayers, their belief in me was not for naught and I added the words that would eventually become the title of this book, *"I'm Not Done Yet."* Because as I've said before, I'm not.

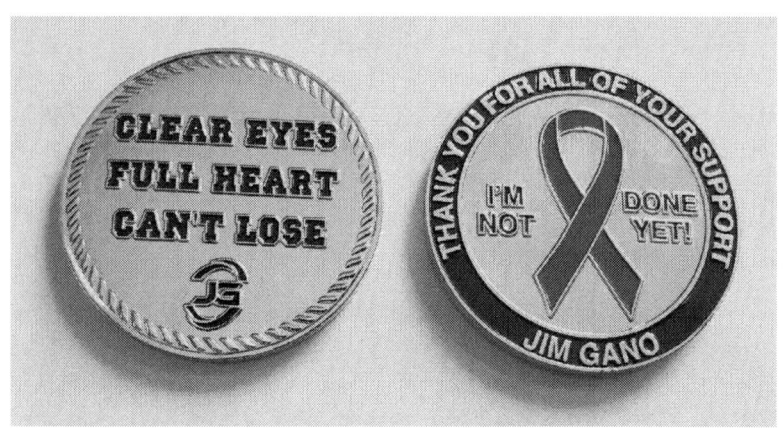

My Challenge Coin I designed for Doctors, Nurses, Family & Friends as a thank you.

Every day as I get ready to leave the house I go through the same routine, wallet, pens, keys, phone and challenge coin. I carry it with me wherever I go. It serves me in many ways. First, as a reminder of where I've been and all I went through. Second, it calms me when the 'little gray cloud' tries to force its way into my brain. All I have to do is either put my hand in my pocket and touch the coin, or take it out and rub my fingers over it and read the messages and

I am okay again.

When I come home at night, I take everything out of my pockets and the last thing I do is place the coin front side up so the phrase Clear Eyes, Full Heart, Can't Lose is the first thing I see the next time I need to go somewhere.

This may seem trivial, but it works for me. Many people on the Multiple Myeloma forum board have told me that they love my mantra phrase, some have even told me they have started using it for themselves.

Since I handed these out, I have been around people and seen them on their desks, in their purses, one man had it framed with a picture he had taken years ago of us together.

I had a few questions about my follow up care and left a message one night on the nurse's line at the hospital where I had my transplant performed. I was concerned when they didn't call back right away. At 7:30p.m. that night the doctor who leads the entire transplant department called me herself to answer my questions, then she spent ten minutes thanking me for her coin. She also said, "I get a lot of gifts from patients and I appreciate them all, but yours is the only one that is now prominently displayed on my desk." I thought that was pretty cool.

My other favorite story is from a nurse named Gail who had to sit with me for three of the five days it took to collect my cells for the Stem cell transplant. She would monitor my vitals and the machine that was extracting the cells. This took about 8–9 hours every day so we talked. A lot.

We talked about our families, work, cancer, the hospital I was being treated in and she really calmed me down and made me feel like I was in good hands. We talked about my writing and I gave her a copy of my book *"The Player,"* which she not only read, but has shared with many of her friends and colleagues. In effect, we really got to know each other, and her "daughter", (a fellow nurse she calls daughter, but that is a story for another time). Those two are too cute together.

Every time I have a follow up appointment Gail makes sure she is on the schedule to work and she makes sure to stop by while I am getting my vaccines so we can catch up. As she walks toward me, she either says "I still have my coin," or she pulls it out of her pocket to show me.

Be different to be remembered.

All of these people are special to me and I always tried to learn a little something about each one. Many times, patients meet with doctors and become mutes. Just answering questions, but never getting to know the person(s) responsible for their care. Ask them questions. Do they have any dogs or cats? Are they Giants or Jets fans? Do they have any interests outside of work? Do they wear boxers or briefs? No wait a minute scratch that last one, that may be too much information.

I am not a big fan of soccer. I liked to play it as a kid, I coached my son's recreation soccer team to an overall record of 130-0-3, but I don't sit down on a Sunday afternoon to watch a match. But my Oncologist travelled halfway around the world to see the World Cup last time it was played so now I had something I could talk to him about. My Nurse Practitioner just had a baby so I always ask to see updated photo's. What Mom wouldn't want to show you a picture of her baby?

Make connections so that you have something other than cancer to talk about. When discussing marketing with my clients I always say "we are trying to create a 'front of mind' presence with your customers and potential customers." The same is true of your doctor's. I want them thinking of me long after they've left my treatment room so they are making sure I am receiving the best treatment available then.

It's funny because some doctor's when they hear of my background have actually called me to see if I can refer someone I know for a service they need.

I'm not saying you will develop this relationship with your team, but it doesn't hurt.

Motivational Quotes

Here are some of my favorite motivational quotes that when I need a little extra motivation can get me going. Where possible I have given credit to the author. Maybe you can use them as well if you need that little push occasionally.

**"Never let it rest,
until your good is better,
and your better is best."
James E. Gano, Jr. (My Dad)**

**"The difference between ordinary
and extraordinary
is that little <u>EXTRA</u>."**

"TNT – <u>T</u>oday <u>N</u>ot <u>T</u>omorrow"
Larry Winget

**"Throw me to the wolves,
and I'll return leading the pack."**

-----

*"It is not the critic who counts; not the man
who points out how the strong man stumbles,
or where the doer of deeds could have done
them better. The credit belongs to the man who
is actually in the arena, whose face is marred
by dust and sweat and blood; who strives
valiantly; who errs, who comes short again and
again, because there is no effort without error
and shortcoming; but who does actually strive
to do the deeds; who knows great enthusiasms,
the great devotions; who spends himself in a
worthy cause; who at the best knows in the end
the triumph of high achievement, and who at
the worst, if he fails, at least fails while daring
greatly, so that his place shall never be with
those cold and timid souls who neither know
victory nor defeat."*
Teddy Roosevelt

**The Devil whispered in my ear,
"You're not ready for the storm."
"I whispered back, *I am the storm*."**

"Power Through It."
Me

"The windshield is so much bigger than the rearview mirror because there is so much in front of you instead of what's behind you."

"Don't give up. Don't ever give up."
Jim Valvano

"You must make a goal for yourself.
Once you accomplish this goal, you are not done.
You must make another and ... GO FOR IT!"
Jim Gano (Also Me)

To all the doors that closed on me:
I'm coming back to buy the building.

REFUSE TO LOSE!
Ray Evernham

"You never lose, if you never quit"

"I haven't had a bad day since the doctor slapped me on the ass!"
Jon Bon Jovi

-----

*"Live your life each day as you
would climb a mountain.
An occasional glance toward the
summit keeps the goal in mind,
but many beautiful scenes
are to be observed from each new
vantage point.
Climb slowly, steadily, enjoying
each passing moment; and the view
from the summit will serve as a
fitting climax for the journey."*
Harold V. Melchert

-----

*"Life is a harsh teacher,
it gives you the grade first,
and the lesson later."*
Ann Landers

"Never, Never, Never Quit."
Winston Churchill

-----

*"You may encounter many defeats,
but you must not be defeated."*
Maya Angelou

-----

*"You're braver than you believe, stronger
than you seem, and smarter than you think."*
Christopher Robin to Winnie the Pooh

This is one of my favorite poems I used often when I was either physically or emotionally spent during treatment.

Don't Quit

When things go wrong, as they sometimes will,
when the road you're trudging seems all uphill,
when the funds are low and the debts are high,
and you want to smile but you have to sigh,
when care is pressing you down a bit –
rest if you must, but don't you quit.

Life is queer with its twists and turns.
As everyone of us sometimes learns.
And many a fellow turns about,
when he might have won had he stuck it out.
Don't give up though the pace seems slow -
you may succeed with another blow.
Often the goal is nearer than it seems to a faint
and faltering man;

Often the struggler has given up
when he might have captured the victor's cup;
and he learned too late when the night came
down, how close he was to the golden crown.

Success is failure turned inside out -
the silver tint of the clouds of doubt,
and when you never can tell how close you are,
it may be near when it seems afar;
so stick to the fight when you're hardest hit -
it's when things seem worst, you must not quit.

The Dash by Linda Ellis

I read of a man who stood to speak at the funeral
of a friend.
He referred to the dates on the tombstone from
the beginning to the end.
He noted first came the date of the birth and
spoke the following date with tears.
But he said what mattered most of all was the
dash between the years.
For that dash represents all the time
that they spent life on Earth.
And now only those who loved them know what
that little line is worth.
For it matters not how much we own,
the cars, the house, the cash.
What matters is how we live and love,
and how we spend our dash.
So, think about this long and hard.
Are there things you'd like to change?
For you never know how much time is left that
can still be rearranged.
If we could just slow down enough
to consider what's true and real,
and always try to understand
the way other people feel.
And be less quick to anger,
and show appreciation more,
and love the people in our lives
like we've never loved before.
If we treat each other with respect
and more often wear a smile,
remembering that this special dash
might only last a little while.
So, when your eulogy is being read with your
life's actions to rehash,
would you be proud of the things they say about
how you spent your dash?

Final thoughts

Well, there you have it, some of my thoughts of what it took for me to beat cancer ... for now. My type of cancer I am told will return at some point, which I hope is a long time away from now. I do know that with my mindset I will meet it head on if it ever decides to return. Remember, I have to go to my Grandson's wedding.

My hope with this book is that I motivated or inspired you in some way to keep fighting, and never give up. I hope that you are a fighter and that you will do *whatever it takes'* to beat this invisible foe, cancer.

If you are a cancer patient, I hope that my story shows that you can not only survive, but thrive with this diagnosis. It is my sincerest hope and prayer, that you will have a positive outcome from your care and treatments. And please remember to treat those caring for you with love, care and respect. If you get the chance to ring that bell, ring the hell out of it so I can hear it all the way here in New Jersey. Ring it for everyone who couldn't ring the bell, as well as for yourself.

For the caregiver, I want to start with a very simple, *thank you.* You have one of the toughest jobs on the planet caring for someone you love at a time when they are at their lowest. I know it isn't easy and I hope that they appreciate all you do for them as much as I did my wife caring for me. Remember, sometimes the drugs can mess with their brains and affect their personality and that sweet person you once knew and loved, can become someone you barely recognize for the way they speak to you, or treat you. It is not your fault. Unfortunately, you are the one that they will lash out at. Please don't take it personally, but do remind them that you are there for them, and deserve better consideration. Ask them to 'find their neutral.' The sooner in the process you have this discussion, the more mindful they will be when dealing with you.

Nobody asks to get cancer. One person in the hospital said to me, "welcome to the club" as we were getting our weekly dose of chemo. I told her, "This is one club I have no desire to join."

As mentioned in an earlier chapter you will probably have to process the five stages of grief but to me the sooner you get to the 'acceptance' stage, meaning you acknowledge you have cancer, the sooner you can be on the road to recovery, or better yet, remission.

Every form of cancer is different, so I don't

mean to minimize the battle you will go through. Nor did I try to make it sound like mine was easy, it was not. As I told my wife as we drove home from the hospital on my birthday after the Stem cell transplant as I broke down and cried with tears in my eyes, this was the hardest thing I have ever done.

For some, cancer is caught early and they go through treatment and they move on. For others, the fight will be harder either due to when the disease was discovered, or the type of cancer they have, or the stage they are in. Regardless of that, I ask that you find your 'why' and fight for that reason. It might be your family, your children, yourself, your business, your dog or cat. Whatever the reason, whatever your why, have that *Man in the Arena* mentality that Teddy Roosevelt talks about. When you fight, fight like I did with this mentality:

Clear Eyes.
Full Heart.
Can't Lose.

As for me, I don't know what the future holds. My cancer, my little gray cloud, could come back tomorrow, or it could wait ten years or more. I assure you that you will not find me sitting on the sidelines waiting for it. I will be out there living my life, running my business, playing with my grandchildren, driving my 1948 Plymouth Special Deluxe (with a big old smile on my face when I do), enjoying as much time as I can with my wife, my family and my friends, travelling, learning new things, announcing football and basketball games at the local high school and the list goes on and on. I'll be filling *my* dash.

Mine has been a life well lived, and I am grateful for every minute I have had the blessing to live it.

You can bet that if someone asks me to do something, I'll probably do it. (Except jump out of an airplane). I will continue to try to help those less fortunate than me for as long as I can, whether it is the students in the Workplace Readiness Program, or others.

My hope is that I will have many more sunsets to see, and many more days to put to rest, knowing I have gotten as much out of that day as I possibly could.

I will live. I will live my life the way I always have, by getting involved and trying to make a difference in the lives of those around me. And I will do all this for as long as I humanly can. I also hope this book and these thoughts have made a difference in your life. I hope that when I'm gone at some point someone stops and thinks of me and says, *"he made a difference in my life."*

I also hope that I have many more productive years here on earth to do just that.

All I know is, ***"I'm Not Done Yet!"***

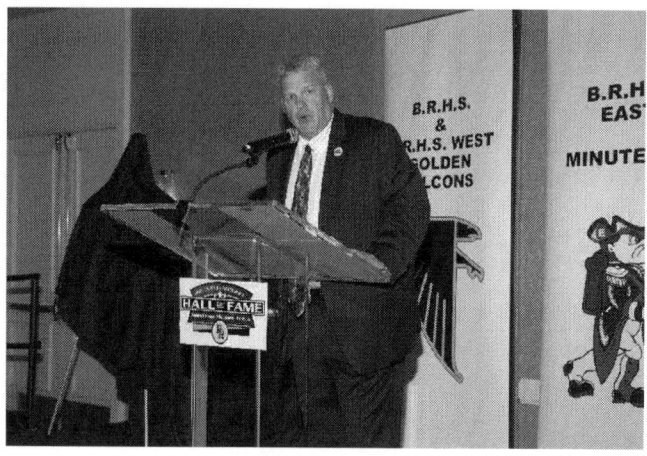

The author being inducted into the Bridgewater-Raritan High
School Athletic Hall of Fame – October 5, 2024

The End

Well, not really, more like the beginning.

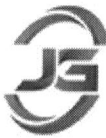

About the Author

Jim Gano was born and raised and still lives in his hometown of Bridgewater, New Jersey. He has been very active in his community over the years having served on the local rescue squad and getting involved in issues that directly affect the people of Bridgewater.

For over forty-two years, Jim has served as *"The Voice"* of Bridgewater-Raritan High School Athletics and has served on numerous committees at the school that have benefitted the students and athletes there. In 2024 Jim was inducted into the school's Athletic Hall of Fame for his efforts.

Jim is the owner of the multiple award-winning Crown Trophy of Flemington and Signs By Crown of Flemington franchises, a local awards retailer and sign shop that he has owned and run for over fifteen years.

Jim is also a published author having two books in the fiction genre, *"The Student"* and *"The Player"* published to critical acclaim.

He has served on numerous boards in his community with the goal of making these organizations and the people they serve better than when he joined them.

Jim hosts a weekly radio show/podcast on Thursdays on Hunterdon Chamber Radio called "Takin' Care of Business with Jim Gano" where he discusses issues and trends that affect small businesses.

Jim has been married to his wife Carol for 38 years and together they have two children along with their respective wife and fiancée and three Grandchildren whom he adores.

Jim recently joined "The Cancer Hope Network" where he serves as a volunteer peer mentor helping guide newly diagnosed patients on their journey with cancer.

Jim is often asked to speak to corporations and local organizations to spread his message of inspiration and hope and to motivate others to 'get involved.' If you would like Jim to speak to your organization, or book club, either in person or online via Zoom, contact him at the email address below.

Did you enjoy this book? Let the author know by sending an email to: jegthe3@gmail.com.

If you enjoyed this book the publisher asks that you please leave a review by the book's title "I'm Not Done Yet" by Jim Gano on Amazon.com

For more information about the author visit his website at www.jimgano.com

I'm Not Done Yet

Made in United States
Orlando, FL
05 December 2025